Curbside Consultation
of the Colon

49 Clinical Questions

CURBSIDE CONSULTATION IN GASTROENTEROLOGY
SERIES

SERIES EDITOR, FRANCIS A. FARRAYE, MD, MSc

Curbside
Consultation
of the Colon

49 Clinical Questions

EDITED BY

Brooks D. Cash, MD, FACP, FACG
Chief
Gastroenterology Division and Colon Health Initiative
National Naval Medical Center
Associate Professor, USUHS
Bethesda, MD

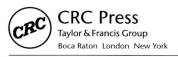

CRC Press
Taylor & Francis Group
Boca Raton London New York

CRC Press is an imprint of the
Taylor & Francis Group, an **informa** business

First published 2009 by SLACK Incorporated

Published 2024 by CRC Press
2385 NW Executive Center Drive, Suite 320, Boca Raton FL 33431

and by CRC Press
4 Park Square, Milton Park, Abingdon, Oxon, OX14 4RN

CRC Press is an imprint of Taylor & Francis Group, LLC

Library of Congress Cataloging-in-Publication Data

Curbside consultation of the colon : 49 clinical questions / edited by Brooks D. Cash.
    p. ; cm. -- (Curbside consultation in gastroenterology)
    Includes bibliographical references and index.
    ISBN 978-1-55642-831-9 (alk. paper)
    1. Colon (Anatomy)--Diseases--Miscellanea. I. Cash, Brooks D., 1967- II. Series.
    [DNLM: 1. Colonic Diseases. WI 520 C975 2008]
    RC860.C83 2008
    616.3'4--dc22
                                2008030255

ISBN: 9781556428319 (pbk)
ISBN: 9781003523734 (ebk)

DOI: 10.1201/9781003523734

Dedication

To Marianne, Madison, and Grayson. Thank you for your patience and support and for keeping the home fires burning.

Contents

Acknowledgments

The author would like to acknowledge the following individuals for their dedication and help with this book: Carrie Kotlar, Philip Schoenfeld, Brian Lacy, Arnie Wald, Inku Hwang, Scott Itzkowitz, Brennan Spiegel, Richard Saad, Brian Mulhall, and, most of all, Francis Farraye.

About the Editor

Brooks D. Cash, MD, FACP, FACG is the Chief of Gastroenterology and the Colon Health Initiative at the National Naval Medical Center in Bethesda, Maryland. Dr. Cash received his medical degree from the Uniformed Services University of Medicine (USUHS) in Bethesda, and completed his internal medicine residency and gastroenterology fellowship training at the National Naval Medical Center. Board certified in gastroenterology, he currently serves as an Associate Professor of Medicine at USUHS. Active in research, his main areas of interest are wide ranging and consist primarily of functional gastrointestinal disorders, acid peptic disorders, and colorectal cancer screening. He currently oversees multiple ongoing protocols in all of these areas and, as a leader in the field of CT colonography, he currently oversees multiple studies designed to clarify and expand the practice of this new technology. He is the author of numerous book chapters, review articles, and peer-reviewed manuscripts; is actively involved in committee work for various gastroenterology professional societies; and serves on the editorial boards of multiple professional journals.

Contributing Authors

B. Joe Elmunzer, MD (Question 2)
Division of Gastroenterology
Department of Medicine
University of Michigan Medical Center
Ann Arbor, MI

Francis A. Farraye, MD, MSc (Questions 8, 10, 11)
Clinical Director, Section of Gastroenterology
Boston Medical Center
Professor of Medicine
Boston University School of Medicine
Boston, MA

Christopher S. Huang, MD (Questions 10, 11)
Boston Medical Center
Assistant Professor of Medicine
Boston University School of Medicine
Boston, MA

Inku Hwang, MD (Questions 40-44)
Staff Gastroenterologist
Wenatchee Valley Medical Center
Wenatchee, WA

Scott L. Itzkowitz, DO, FACP (Questions 45-49)
Staff Gastroenterologist
Director of Endoscopy
Assistant Professor of Medicine
F. Edward Hebert School of Medicine
Uniformed Services University of the Health Sciences
National Naval Medical Center
Bethesda, MD

Brian E. Lacy, MD, PhD (Questions 31-34, 36-39)
Associate Professor of Medicine
Director of Gastroenterology and Hepatology
Dartmouth-Hitchcock Medical Center
Lebanon, NH

L. Campbell Levy, MD (Question 35)
Assistant Professor of Medicine
Dartmouth Medical School
Dartmouth-Hitchcock Medical Center
Lebanon, NH

Brian Mulhall, MD (Questions 21, 22, 24-26)
Tacoma Digestive Disease Center
Tacoma, WA

Michael J. O'Brien, MD, MPH (Questions 10, 11)
Chief of Anatomic Pathology
Boston Medical Center
Professor of Pathology and Laboratory Medicine
Boston University School of Medicine
Boston, MA

Erica Roberson, MD (Questions 12-18)
Women's Health Fellow
William S. Middleton Memorial VA Medical Center
University of Wisconsin Hospital & Clinics
Madison, WI

Richard Saad, MD (Questions 20, 27-29)
Clinical Lecturer
Division of Gastroenterology
Department of Internal Medicine
University of Michigan Health System
Ann Arbor, MI

Philip Schoenfeld, MD, MSEd, MSc (Epi) (Questions 1-3)
Veterans Affairs Center for Excellence in Health Services Research
Veterans Administration Medical Center
Ann Arbor, MI

Corey A. Siegel, MD (Question 35)
Assistant Professor of Medicine,
Dartmouth Medical School Director,
Inflammatory Bowel Disease Center,
Dartmouth-Hitchcock Medical Center
Lebanon, NH

Amit Singal, MD (Question 3)
Division of Gastroenterology
University of Michigan
Ann Arbor, MI

Inder Singh, MD (Questions 4, 5)
Fellow-Gastroenterology
UCLA Division of Digestive Diseases
Los Angeles, CA

Brennan Spiegel, MD, MSHS (Questions 4, 5)
Assistant Professor of Medicine
VA Greater Los Angeles Healthcare
    System
David Geffen School of Medicine at UCLA
Chief of Education and Training, UCLA GI
    Fellowship Program
Director, UCLA/VA Center for Outcomes
    Research and Education (CORE)
Los Angeles, CA

Jason Taylor, MD (Question 1)
Division of Gastroenterology
Department of Medicine
University of Michigan Medical Center
Ann Arbor, MI

Arnold Wald, MD (Questions 12-18)
Professor, Section of Gastroenterology
Department of Internal Medicine
School of Medicine & Public Health
University of Wisconsin Hospital & Clinics
Madison, WI

Preface

Much of the field of gastroenterology centers on care of disorders of the colon. This remarkable organ continues to fascinate clinicians and patients alike. From inflammatory diseases, to infections, to malignancies, to functional disorders, the precise workings of the colon, and the origins of the disorders that affect it, are still not completely understood. It is remarkable that in 2008, fallacies and misconceptions about how the colon functions still abound. We created this book to address many of these misconceptions. We also wrote it to answer commonly posed questions, and to do so based on the latest clinical evidence. To accomplish that goal, I was fortunate enough to have a dedicated group of expert clinicians and researchers willing to share their expertise and time to answer these questions. These experts have been able to concisely summarize difficult concepts into easily understood and retained answers that the interested reader will be able to use in his or her clinical practice, either in the direct treatment of specific patients, patient counseling, or the mentoring of colleagues and trainees.

Foreword

The intrigue for the specialty of Gastroenterology is, in part, due to the broad knowledge of pathology and physiology that must be drawn upon in order to make a proper diagnosis. The satisfaction in caring for an individual with a digestive disease comes from the ability to recognize the disorder and tailor an optimal treatment strategy for each patient. Whether it is in the outpatient or inpatient setting, acute and chronic colonic symptoms and disorders make up a large majority of the caseload of the patients evaluated by a digestive disease specialist each day. A busy clinician will find it difficult to maintain the knowledge base needed for the care of his or her patient without an excellent external resource.

A portion of the vast wealth of knowledge required to stay abreast of the current management of colonic diseases has been culled into a handy reference book by Brooks Cash, MD. Dr. Cash has assembled a group of expert contributors in *Curbside Consultation of the Colon* to pose 49 of the most pertinent and frequently seen clinical scenarios. The answers are concise and easily readable. All clinicians will find extremely useful the information on the utility and rationale for colorectal cancer screening and chemoprevention, and strategies for the management of sporadic and hereditary colorectal neoplasms. The experts' recommendations for the diagnostic evaluation and treatment of patients with both constipation and diarrhea is well covered. The clinical scenarios posed review the treatment strategies for common clinical conundrums such as the management of individuals with both active IBD and concomitant *Clostridium difficile* infection, and the evidence for the use of antibiotics in IBS or as prophylaxis for endoscopic procedures. Practical tips for the management of the commonly seen perianal disorders such as proctalgia fugax, fissures and hemorrhoids are nicely incorporated among other, more varied subjects such as Ogilvie's syndrome, pneumatosis coli, diverticular disease, and the effects of NSAIDS on the colon.

Individuals at all levels of training and practice will find *Curbside Consultation of the Colon* a welcome addition to their library.

Carol Burke, MD
Director, Center for Colon Polyps & Cancer
Department of Gastroenterology
Cleveland Clinics
Cleveland, Ohio

Introduction

We wrote this book for the busy clinician. Appropriate for both specialists and primary care providers, the book is designed to serve as a ready guide to provide answers for some of the most commonly asked or encountered questions and clinical scenarios involving the colon. Conceptually, the book is divided into several sections that address general areas of colonic function and dysfunction. The first section of the book deals with the evolving field of colorectal cancer and provides the reader with up-to-date guidance on screening and surveillance recommendations for a variety of patients, while also delving into the more esoteric subjects of inherited cancer syndromes and the interpretation of pathologic descriptions of different types of polyps. The following two sections cover topics within the symptomatic extremes of constipation and diarrhea. Topics such as melanosis coli, irritable bowel syndrome, infectious diarrhea, and inflammatory bowel disease are among the subjects discussed in these sections. These are followed by a section focused on the diagnosis and treatment of a variety of perianal disorders such as strictures and hemorrhoids, incredibly common disorders that are among the most bothersome to our patients. Finally, the last series of curbside consultations addresses a number of other commonly encountered clinical questions and scenarios such as the diagnosis and management of colonic pseudo-obstruction and diverticulitis, to name a few. The overarching goal of this book is to provide a ready reference to commonly asked questions and, to this end, I believe we have succeeded. The expert contributors to the book have delivered a concise, easy-to-use reference that will be welcome in the lab coat pocket, the desk, or within ready reach in the bookcase. I hope that the reader enjoys using it as much as we enjoyed writing it.

SECTION I

COLON CANCER SCREENING

A 46-YEAR-OLD AFRICAN AMERICAN MAN WHO HAS NO ALARM FEATURES OR SYMPTOMS REQUESTS A SCREENING COLONOSCOPY. IS THIS APPROPRIATE?

Jason Taylor, MD
Philip Schoenfeld, MD, MSEd, MSc (Epi)

Colonoscopy is the gold standard screening tool for colorectal cancer, and it is offered routinely to average risk individuals older than 50 years. However, there has been an ongoing debate about whether this standard recommendation should be altered for African Americans, with colonoscopy offered to average-risk African Americans older than 45 years.[1] The issue remains controversial with data to support and refute this recommendation.

The impetus for this debate began in the 1990s when data identified race related variability in colorectal cancer incidence and survival. The debate heightened in 2002 after the Institute of Medicine issued a report that stressed racial disparities in health care.[2] Subsequently, greater emphasis was placed on evaluating colorectal cancer with race-specific data, and investigators found epidemiologic data to suggest race disparity for colorectal cancer incidence and survival since 1975.[3]

In 1975, the Surveillance, Epidemiology, and End Results program (SEER database) was started by the National Cancer Institute. This database includes colorectal cancer incidence and survival rates separated by race from 1975 to 2003. Upon review of the colorectal cancer incidence rates from 1996 to 2000, there was a 12.3% higher incidence of colorectal cancer for African Americans as a group when compared to Caucasians.[3] This elevated incidence rate is seen in African Americans age 46 to 50 when compared to their Caucasian counterparts at the same age. Although there is no clear explanation for this difference, several studies have suggested that lower use of diagnostic testing and variability in screening rates are confounding factors.[4-7]

In addition to the increased incidence of colorectal cancer among African Americans, the SEER database also demonstrated a discrepancy in survival after diagnosis of colorectal cancer. The 5-year survival rate for colorectal cancer among African Americans was 53% from 1992 to 1999, whereas Caucasians had a 63% survival rate.[3] Several experts state that access to health care, less use of diagnostic tests, and lower screening rates could account for this difference.[5,6,8,9] Regardless, the discrepancies in both incidence and survival served as the impetus for the American College of Gastroenterology (ACG) to comment on this topic in 2005.

In March 2005, the ACG Committee of Minority Affairs and Cultural Diversity published its report on this topic. After reviewing the current research regarding colorectal cancer in African Americans, the committee members recommended that colorectal cancer screening with colonoscopy should begin at age 45 in average-risk African Americans.[1] This was the first time that a gastrointestinal or cancer society favored a change in colorectal cancer screening guidelines based on race alone. Even though the article was widely publicized, there has not been a change in the consensus recommendation for colorectal cancer screening in average-risk individuals by either the American Gastroenterological Association or the American Cancer Society. Both societies continue to recommend that screening for colorectal cancer begin at age 50.[10,11]

Currently, we lack data from well-designed population-based trials about the incidence of colon adenomas and colorectal cancer among Caucasians, African Americans, Hispanics, and Asians. It is possible that the differences observed in African Americans result from differences in access to health care or other confounding factors that are poorly understood. In fact, a recent meta-analysis found a pooled hazard ratio for colon cancer-specific mortality to be only marginally higher in African Americans when compared to Caucasians. The study concludes that there is no strong evidence for racial disparities in colorectal cancer survival after accounting for racial differences in socioeconomic status.[12] Moreover, one study done at a US Veterans Health Care System showed no survival difference in African Americans and Caucasians with colorectal cancer.[13] This study supports the notion that equal access to health care negates racial discrepancies in survival with regard to colorectal cancer.

Until more definitive evidence for a change in screening guidelines emerges, we recommend the patient in this clinical scenario wait until age 50 for his colonoscopy. Of course, if the patient has any "danger" signs, such as hematochezia or unexplained weight loss, then colonoscopy should be performed immediately. We also support the recommendations of the Institute of Medicine and the ACG for further research in this area. Finally, greater efforts should be made to ensure that all average-risk individuals get colorectal cancer screening starting at age 50.

References

1. Agrawal S, Bhupinderjit A, Bhutani MS, et al. Committee of Minority Affairs and Cultural Diversity, American College of Gastroenterology. Colorectal cancer in African Americans. *Am J Gastroenterol.* 2005;100(3):515-523.
2. Institute of Medicine. *Unequal Treatment: Confronting Racial and Ethnic Disparities in Health Care.* Washington, DC: National Academy Press; 2002.
3. Rise LAG, Eisner MP, Kosary CL, et al, eds. *SEER Cancer Statistics Review, 1975-2000.* Bethesda, MD. National Cancer Institute. Available at: http://seer.cancer.gov/csr/1975_2000. Accessed June 2, 2008.

4. Coughlin SS, Thompson TD, Seeff L, et al. Breast, cervical, and colorectal carcinoma screening in a demographically defined region of the southern U.S. *Cancer.* 2002;95(10):2211-2222.
5. Ioannou GN, Chapko MK, Dominitz JA. Predictors of colorectal cancer screening participation in the United States. *Am J Gastroenterol.* 2003;98(9):2082-2091.
6. Richards RJ, Reker DM. Racial differences in use of colonoscopy, sigmoidoscopy, and barium enema in Medicare beneficiaries. *Dig Dis Sci.* 2002;47(12):2715-2719.
7. McMahon LF Jr, Wolfe RA, Huang S, Tedeschi P, Manning W Jr, Edlund MJ. Racial and gender variation in use of diagnostic colonic procedures in the Michigan Medicare population. *Med Care.* 1999;37(7):712-717.
8. Marcella S, Miller JE. Racial differences in colorectal cancer mortality: the importance of stage and socioeconomic status. *J Clin Epidemiol.* 2001;54(4):359-366.
9. Roetzheim RG, Pal N, Gonzalez EC, Ferrante JM, Van Durme DJ, Krischer JP. Effects of health insurance and race on colorectal cancer treatments and outcomes. *Am J Public Health.* 2000;90(11):1746-1754.
10. Winawer S, Fletcher R, Rex D, et al. Colorectal cancer screening and surveillance: clinical guidelines and rationale—update based on new evidence. *Gastroenterology.* 2003;124(2):544-560.
11. American Cancer Society. *Cancer Facts & Figures 2007.* Atlanta, Ga: American Cancer Society; 2007.
12. Du XL, Meyer TE, Franzini L. Meta-analysis of racial disparities in survival in association with socioeconomic status among men and women with colon cancer. *Cancer.* 2007;109(11):2161-2170.
13. Dominitz JA, Samsa GP, Landsman P, Provenzale D. Race, treatment, and survival among colorectal carcinoma patients in an equal-access medical system. *Cancer.* 1998;82(12):2312-2320.

What Pathologic Analysis Do I Need to Pursue in a 38-Year-Old Man With Cecal Cancer Whose Family History Is Suspicious for Hereditary Nonpolyposis Colon Cancer?

B. Joe Elmunzer, MD
Philip Schoenfeld, MD, MSEd, MSc (Epi)

Colorectal cancer (CRC) is a preventable malignancy that ranks fourth worldwide in both incidence and cancer-related deaths. Advanced age is a powerful predictor of CRC: more than 90% of patients are older than 50 years at the time of diagnosis. In patients who develop CRC at a younger age (<50 years), there is a reasonable probability that the malignancy has developed as part of a familial colon cancer syndrome.[1] The most common hereditary colon cancer syndromes are listed in Table 2-1.

Hereditary nonpolyposis colon cancer (HNPCC) is characterized by early-onset cancers occurring primarily in the colon and female reproductive system. Patients with HNPCC who develop colon cancer are more likely to have right-sided (proximal) colon cancers, so screening should be performed with colonoscopy. The best defined form of HNPCC is Lynch syndrome, an autosomal dominant defect in mismatch repair genes that renders them ineffective at protecting the genetic code from potentially carcinogenic mutations. This failure results in the phenomenon of microsatellite instability (MSI) in which short, repeated DNA sequences become susceptible to somatic mutation by misalignment.[2] Only 55% of families that meet criteria for HNPCC will actually have Lynch syndrome. The remainder of cases designated familial colorectal cancer type X do not have DNA mismatch repair gene defects as the etiology of their malignancies.[3] The Amsterdam criteria for the diagnosis of HNPCC are listed in Table 2-2.

Table 2-1

Hereditary Colorectal Cancer Syndromes

- Hereditary nonpolyposis colon cancer
- Familial adenomatous polyposis (including attenuated FAP)
- Gardner's syndrome
- MYH-associated polyposis
- Peutz-Jehgers syndrome
- Juvenile polyposis syndrome

Table 2-2

Amsterdam II Criteria for Diagnosing HNPCC

- At least 3 relatives have a cancer associated with HNPCC (CRC, cancer of the endometrium, small bowel, or renal pelvis)
- One relative should be a first-degree relative of the other 2 relatives
- At least 2 successive generations should be affected
- At least 1 relative should be diagnosed before the age of 50 years
- FAP should be excluded
- Tumors should be verified by pathologic examination

Adapted from Vasen HF, Watson P, Mecklin JP, Lynch HT. New clinical criteria for hereditary nonpolyposis colorectal cancer (HNPCC, Lynch syndrome) proposed by the International Collaborative group on HNPCC. *Gastroenterology.* 1999;116(6):1453-1456.

Table 2-3

Management Guidelines for At-risk Members of Families With Lynch Syndrome (Hereditary Mismatch Repair Gene Mutation)

- Intitial colonoscopy at age 20 to 25, or 10 years before the youngest age at diagnosis in a relative (whichever comes first)
- Colonoscopy every 1 to 2 years thereafter
- Endometrial sampling yearly starting at age 30 to 35
- Transvaginal ultrasound yearly starting at age 30 to 35
- Urinalysis with cytology every 1 to 2 years starting at age 25 to 35

Adapted from Lindor N, Petersen G, Hadley D, et al. Recommendations for the care of individuals with an inherited predisposition to Lynch syndrome: a systematic review. *JAMA.* 2006;296(12):1507-1517.

When managing a young patient (<50 years) with CRC, attention should always be paid to the possibility of an inherited colon cancer syndrome, particularly if the patient has a personal or family history of compatible malignancies (see Table 2-2). Diagnosing such a familial syndrome has major implications in future malignancy screening for both the patient and his relatives. The most widely recommended screening strategy for families with HNPCC is outlined in Table 2-3.[4]

In this patient, the resected CRC specimen should be submitted to a specialized laboratory for MSI and immunohistochemistry testing. The presence of either MSI or demonstrated loss of HNPCC-related protein products through immunohistochemical analysis secures the diagnosis of Lynch syndrome. This diagnosis should then prompt serum testing for identifiable germline mutations in DNA mismatch repair genes, which will be present in approximately 50% of patients with Lynch syndrome. The presence of these mutations may be helpful in identifying family members with Lynch syndrome who require aggressive screening.[5]

If MSI is absent (or low) and/or immunohistochemistry demonstrates intact DNA mismatch repair proteins in the surgical specimen, then Lynch syndrome is very unlikely. If the patient's family, however, fulfills pedigree criteria for HNPCC, then a diagnosis of familial colorectal cancer type X can be made. Such patients appear to be at higher risk for CRC than the general population, although at lower risk than those with Lynch syndrome. The optimal screening for this patient population has not yet been defined.

If the patient's family does not fulfill strict criteria for HNPCC and his CRC specimen is negative for both MSI and immunohistochemical evidence of protein product loss, then an inherited colorectal cancer syndrome is unlikely, and first-degree relatives should begin colorectal cancer screening with colonoscopy at age 28 (10 years younger than the index patient who is 38 years old) with repeat colonoscopy every 3 to 5 years depending on whether or not adenomas are identified.

All patients who are diagnosed with CRC at a young age benefit from evaluation by a medical geneticist as the decision-making process is complex and clinical management cannot be based solely on phenotypic evaluation of the tumor or genetic testing.

References

1. Winawer S, Fletcher R, Miller L, et al. AGA guidelines: colorectal cancer screening: clinical guidelines and rationale. *Gastroenterology*. 1997;112(2):594-642.
2. Jass J, Cottier D, Jeevaratnam P, et al. Diagnostic use of microsatellite instability in hereditary nonpolyposis colorectal cancer. *Lancet*. 1995;346(8984):1200-1201.
3. Lindor NM, Rabe K, Petersen GM, et al. Lower cancer incidence in Amsterdam-I criteria families without mismatch repair deficiency. *JAMA*. 2005;293(16):1979-1985.
4. Lindor N, Petersen G, Hadley D, et al. Recommendations for the care of individuals with an inherited predisposition to Lynch syndrome: a systematic review. *JAMA*. 2006;296(12):1507-1517.
5. American Gastroenterological Association. American Gastroenterological Association medical position statement: hereditary colorectal cancer and genetic testing. *Gastroenterology*. 2001;121(1):195-197.

How Do You Respond to Patients Wanting to Take Aspirin, Calcium, or Other Medications as Prophylaxis for Colorectal Cancer? Is There Any Evidence That They Work?

Amit Singal, MD
Philip Schoenfeld, MD, MSEd, MSc (Epi)

Multiple epidemiological studies have demonstrated an inverse relationship between aspirin use and colorectal cancer. Aspirin, and other NSAIDs, inhibit the COX-2 enzyme, which is highly expressed in colorectal cancer and is involved in inhibition of apoptosis, tumor invasion, and angiogenesis. Thus, aspirin-induced COX-2 inhibition is hypothesized to be the mechanism for aspirin's chemopreventive effect.

Case-control studies demonstrate a wide range of reductions in the relative risk of recurrent adenomas with regular aspirin use. Pooling of the data from these trials showed that aspirin use for less than 3 years is associated with a non-significant trend in favor of aspirin (RR 0.85, 95%, CI 0.72 to 1.0), whereas longer duration of use has a statistically significant effect (RR 0.68, 95%, CI 0.54 to 0.87).[1] Two recent randomized controlled trials confirmed that regular aspirin intake can reduce the rate of recurrent adenomas. In patients with a history of colorectal adenomas, the use of aspirin in doses of 81 to 325 mg daily for at least 1 year resulted in a reduction in the relative rate for recurrent adenomas (RR 0.82, 95%, CI 0.7 to 0.95 for pooled data) compared to non-aspirin-using individuals.

Table 3-1

Agents Studied for Chemoprevention of Colon Cancer

- Aspirin/NSAIDs
- Calcium
- Statins
- Folic acid
- Vitamin B_6
- Ursodiol
- Hormone replacement therapy
- Antioxidants
- Fiber supplements

Although these studies imply that aspirin can be used to prevent recurrent adenomas, there are conflicting data, too. The Physicians' Health Study failed to find a protective effect from 325 mg of aspirin every other day in healthy individuals after 5 years of use. On the other hand, analysis using the Nurses' Health Study found that high doses of aspirin (>14 tablets/week) were associated with a significant reduction in colorectal cancer after at least 10 years of regular use. Although these data are suggestive that higher doses and duration of aspirin use may be necessary, these results reflect our uncertainty about the dose and duration of aspirin use required to prevent adenomas and colorectal cancer.

It remains unclear if aspirin should be routinely implemented for colon polyp prevention. Long-term use of aspirin is associated with substantial gastrointestinal toxicity, and this toxicity increases with higher doses and prolonged use. Clinicians and patients must make individualized decisions based upon an individual's risk for colon cancer, coronary artery disease, and gastrointestinal bleeding and must weigh the likelihood and severity of the potential risks of this approach with the possible benefit.

Calcium has also been considered as another possible chemopreventive agent against colorectal cancer. A pooled analysis of several early epidemiological studies suggested that higher calcium intake was associated with a reduction in the risk of colorectal cancer (RR 0.86, 95%, CI 0.78 to 0.95). A recent Cochrane review found only 2 high-quality randomized controlled trials that evaluated the efficacy of calcium for preventing colon cancer.[2] In one study, subjects with a history of colonic polyps were given 1200 mg of elemental calcium daily and then had a follow-up colonoscopy after a mean duration of 4 years to determine the rate of adenoma recurrence. In the second trial, subjects were given 2000 mg of elemental calcium daily and then had a follow-up colonoscopy after 3 years. When combined, the data from these trials demonstrate a statistically significant reduction of adenomatous polyps in patients receiving calcium (OR 0.74, 95%, CI 0.58 to 0.95). The reader should remember that these trials only included patients with a prior history of adenomas. Hence, these studies assessed the efficacy of calcium for secondary prevention of adenomas, not colon cancer, so it remains unclear how effective calcium supplements would be for primary prevention in the average-risk population.

Other agents, including statins and folic acid, have produced some promising but inconsistent results (Table 3-1). A large case-control study found that statin use for a period of at least 5 years was associated with nearly a 50% relative reduction in the risk of colorectal cancer.[3] Epidemiologic studies have also demonstrated considerable risk reductions for colorectal cancer with folic acid.[4]

References

1. Dube C, Rostom A, Lewin G, et al. The use of aspirin for primary prevention of colorectal cancer: a systematic review prepared for the U.S. Preventive Services Task Force. *Ann Intern Med.* 2007;146(5):365-375.
2. Weingarten MA, Zalmanovici A, Yaphe J. Dietary calcium supplementation for preventing colorectal cancer and adenomatous polyps. *Cochrane Database Syst Rev.* 2005;3:CD003548.
3. Poynter JN, Gruber SB, Higgins PD, et al. Statins and the risk of colorectal cancer. *N Engl J Med.* 2005;352(21):2184-2192.
4. Giovannucci E, Stampfer MJ, Colditz GA, et al. Multivitamin use, folate, and colon cancer in women in the Nurses' Health Study. *Ann Intern Med.* 1998;129(7):517-524.

MY PATIENT HAD A 3-CM SESSILE TUBULOVILLOUS ADENOMA ON THE SIGMOID THAT I REMOVED PIECEMEAL. THE PATHOLOGY LAB CAN'T VERIFY CLEAR MARGIN. WHAT SHOULD I RECOMMEND TO THE PATIENT?

Brennan Spiegel, MD, MSHS
Inder Singh, MD

The main concern here is that your patient has an "advanced adenoma" and that it is unclear whether or not you have obtained sufficient margins on what appeared to be a difficult, piecemeal polypectomy. An advanced adenoma is any polyp that is greater than 1 cm in diameter, that has villous architectural changes (even if it is blended with tubular architecture, as occurred here), or with high-grade dysplasia. In addition, patients with 3 or more adenomas, regardless of size or architecture, are classified as having advanced adenomatous changes. By definition, any adenoma has at least low-grade dysplasia. By size and architecture, this patient clearly has a concerning lesion.

In the absence of high-grade dysplasia, the decision making is not entirely straightforward. One must remain cognizant that there may be residual polyp tissue in the colon and that this lesion's advanced architecture is associated with an increased risk of colon cancer in the future. On the other hand, it seems unlikely (although still possible) that there is frank carcinoma in any remaining polyp tissue, suggesting that surgical resection may not be the optimal management approach. Nonetheless, surgical resection is often considered in patients like this and is usually compared with 2 other options: (1) to resume regular endoscopic surveillance per consensus guidelines (in 3 years given the villous architecture and large polyp size),[1,2] and (2) timely, repeat endoscopy to remove and/or obliterate any remaining tissue, followed by aggressive surveillance.

Each of these strategies has been investigated. Simply returning to regular surveillance, as if this patient were now at average risk for incident colon cancer, is not favorable given the advanced size and architecture of the polyp coupled with the uncertainty of its full resection. Data indicate that polyp or cancer recurrence is as high as 46% over a 3-year period following incomplete resection of large (≥3 cm) sessile lesions.[3] So, you probably should not ignore a "mostly resected" sessile polyp and proceed with regular surveillance.

If you are particularly conservative, or if your patient is particularly concerned or ruminating about the risk of incidental cancer, then you might lean toward surgical resection. At least 1 series indicates that some patients similar to the one in this scenario who are sent for surgical resection do end up with evidence of underlying cancer. Specifically, in a series of 80 patients undergoing surgical resection in the setting of unresectable polyps, 16% were found to have cancer, most of which was fortunately stage I disease (ie, not penetrating the muscularis propria and without nodes or distant spread).[4] It is notable that many patients in this study developed significant postoperative morbidity (38%) and mortality (3%) from surgical intervention. Although these numbers may be higher than the experience at your local facility, they emphasize that surgery is not without its consequences. Decision making must proceed with careful consideration of possible postoperative complications, a thorough discussion between you and your patient about the competing non-surgical options (see below), and establishment of a good relationship between your patient and the consulting surgeon.

The third option of aggressive endoscopic surveillance is currently the most accepted approach for treating cases such as the one presented. In a large prospective study, 302 large polyps (>3 cm) were removed endoscopically.[5] Polyps with high-grade dysplasia or carcinoma were referred for surgery. The rest were followed with repeat endoscopy at 3- to 6-month intervals for 1 year, and then subsequently every 1 to 2 years thereafter. This method proved to be safe and effective. In fact, reviews have shown that with repeated endoscopic treatments (including resection of any residual tissue or argon plasma coagulation [APC] of flat residual tissue), recurrence rates from large resected lesions are as low as 3.8% over 1 to 3 years.[6] In addition, the endoscopist can tattoo the lesion on repeat endoscopy, which serves 2 purposes: (1) it allows the surgeon to more easily identify the lesion should it end up needing resection due to high-grade dysplasia or carcinoma, and (2) it may allow the endoscopist to more easily find the site upon repeat surveillance (if performed within months).

Therefore, in this case, the risk of this incompletely resected polyp should be explained to the patient. I would then have the patient return for repeat endoscopy in a timely interval (days or weeks—not months) with 3 objectives in mind: (1) to perform further piecemeal resection of remaining significant tissue, (2) to obliterate any minor "bumpy" tissue remaining at the site after resection with forceps or snare (eg, using APC), and (3) to consider tattooing the site for ease of subsequent identification. Assuming that histological analysis from repeat resection did not show dysplasia or carcinoma, I would then initiate aggressive surveillance for this patient with follow-up endoscopy every 3 to

6 months for the first year, then every 1 to 3 years thereafter, depending on the incident findings.

References

1. Winawer SJ, Zauber AG, O'Brien MJ, et al. The National Polyp Study. Design, methods, and characteristics of patients with newly diagnosed polyps. The National Polyp Study Workgroup. *Cancer.* 1992;70(5 suppl):1236-1245.
2. Winawer SJ, Zauber AG, Fletcher RH, et al. Guidelines for colonoscopy surveillance after polypectomy: a consensus update by the US Multi-Society Task Force on Colorectal Cancer and the American Cancer Society. *Gastroenterology.* 2006;130(6):1872-1885.
3. Fukami N, Lee JH. Endoscopic treatment of large sessile and flat colorectal lesions. *Curr Opin Gastroenterol.* 2006;22(1):54-59.
4. Alder AC, Hamilton EC, Anthony T, Sarosi GA Jr. Cancer risk in endoscopically unresectable colon polyps. *Am J Surg.* 2006;192(5):644-648.
5. Seitz U, Bohnacker S, Seewald S, Thonke F, Soehendra N. Long-term results of endoscopic removal of large colorectal adenomas. *Endoscopy.* 2003;35(8):S41-S44.
6. Bardan E, Bat L, Melzer E, Shemesh E, Bar-Meir S. Colonoscopic resection of large colonic polyps—a prospective study. Department of Gastroenterology, Chaim Sheba Medical Center, Tel Hashomer, Israel. *Isr J Med Sci.* 1997;33(12):777-780.

THE BOARD OF DIRECTORS OF MY HOSPITAL WANTS TO KNOW THE CURRENT COLORECTAL CANCER SCREENING OPTIONS AND WILL GO WITH WHATEVER I RECOMMEND. WHAT DOES THE EVIDENCE SAY IS THE BEST COLORECTAL CANCER SCREENING REGIMEN?

Brennan Spiegel, MD, MSHS
Inder Singh, MD

There are books written on this topic, so answering this question requires a bit of streamlining. We should start from the premise that colorectal cancer (CRC) screening, in any form, is undoubtedly effective and life saving compared to offering no screening. With the advent of increased age-appropriate CRC screening, patients now receive preventive and therapeutic treatments for this common disease at stages far earlier than ever before.

The current widely available tools for CRC screening include: (1) fecal occult blood testing (FOBT),[1] (2) double contrast barium enema, (3) flexible sigmoidoscopy (flex sig), (4) traditional "optical" colonoscopy, and (5) computed tomography colonography (CTC).[2] For the sake of our discussion, newer tools such as molecular-based fecal tests and pill endoscopy will not be discussed given their limited availability and cost constraints.[3] Of note, the double contrast barium enema is highly dependent on technique and adequate preparation and thus has fallen out of favor. Each of the remaining tests (FOBT, flex sig, optical colonoscopy, CTC) has advantages and disadvantages.

The usual "cage match" of competing options is (1) annual FOBT plus flex sig every 5 years versus (2) optical colonoscopy every 10 years. Guidelines pertaining to virtual colonoscopy are in flux and are discussed at more length below.

Advantages of FOBT plus flex sig include the following: (1) it is accessible to primary care physicians and, thus, easy to enact; (2) it does not require conscious sedation or significant time off from work and, thus, is preferable to some patients; and (3) the up-front costs are lower than colonoscopic approaches (although overall costs might not be). However, there are several notable disadvantages, including: (1) FOBT is not highly sensitive or specific; (2) flex sig leaves more than half the colon uninvestigated—a practice akin to performing mammography on one breast; and (3) flex sig is often uncomfortable for patients, many of whom would prefer a full colonoscopy with sedation.

Optical colonoscopy is generally the most well-accepted screening strategy. Given that the National Polyp Study showed an approximately 10-year continuum from the development of adenomatous polyp to malignancy, regular direct visualization of colonic mucosa every 10 years is a reasonable method for detection and prevention of CRC in average-risk patients. With the addition of annual FOBT, the sensitivity should increase, although this approach has not been tested. Even without FOBT, there is no substitute to directly viewing the colonic mucosa with a camera. This allows a full description of the colonic mucosa, careful evaluation of any identified lesions, and resection of lesions through endoscopic techniques. Currently, no other approach can offer this combination of benefits. However, colonoscopy has notable disadvantages as well, including: (1) it requires advanced training to perform; (2) there is a defined, albeit low, risk of perforation, bleeding, infection, and complications of conscious sedation (all well under 1%); (3) the procedure usually requires conscious sedation, which leads to a missed day of work or other life activities; and (4) up to 10% of the colonic mucosa, particularly areas on the back of folds, cannot be reliably viewed, leading to a defined yet infrequent incidence of missed cancers.

Screening practices in the United States have shown the trend toward increased colonoscopic surveillance over FOBT plus flex sig. In 2000, the American College of Gastroenterology recommended colonoscopy as the preferred tool for CRC screening, given the high sensitivity of the test.[4]

Given the diagnostic and potential therapeutic role of colonoscopy, I would recommend colonoscopy for all average-risk patients starting at age 50 with 10-year intervals. I prefer direct visualization of the colon for routine colorectal cancer screening and would reserve the use of less invasive studies for those patients unwilling to have regular colonoscopic evaluation.

The new tool on the block is CTC, also known as "virtual colonoscopy." This tool, first introduced in the 1990s, has gained growing support for screening of colorectal cancer. CTC currently relies on the use of CT generated 2-dimensional and 3-dimensional reconstructions of the entire colon. Since its inception, the test has grown by leaps and bounds. The test is non-invasive and does not require a physician to perform. In addition, CTC allows assessment of the entire colon, including both mucosal and serosal surfaces, and the entire abdomen. CTC also carries the advantage of reconstructing the entire mucosal surface, which may catch many polyps located on the back of colonic folds, lesions often missed by optical colonoscopy. Some patients may have a preference toward this non-invasive study. In addition, studies have shown that after excluding higher risk patients, widespread use for screening may be cost effective. The test is not without disadvantages. CTC is still inferior to direct optical colonoscopy for the detection of flat lesions or lesions less than 1 cm in size. In addition, CTC needs a tremendously good preparation to avoid false-positive findings. The study is not comfortable to undergo, as the patient's colon will need to undergo insufflation with either air or CO_2 gas. The test takes a significant amount of time for adequate interpretation and requires a trained radiologist for interpretation. However, the test is purely diagnostic and offers no therapeutic effect. Thus, CTC is a useful tool and undoubtedly will take a larger role in CRC screening in the future, but cannot be recommended at this time for widespread routine screening.[5,6]

In the case of patients with increased risk of colorectal cancer (ie, first-degree family relative with adenomas, CRC, personal history of cancer/adenomas, familial adenomatous polyposis, heredity nonpolyposis colorectal cancer, inflammatory bowel disease), colonoscopic screening is the test of choice and should begin at earlier and more aggressive intervals than average colorectal cancer screening. In addition, there is some evidence that screening African Americans at an earlier age may be beneficial.[7]

References

1. Hewitson P, Glasziou P, Irwig L, Towler B, Watson E. Screening for colorectal cancer using the faecal occult blood test, Hemoccult. *Cochrane Database Syst Rev.* 2007;(1):CD001216.
2. Allison JE, Lawson M. Screening tests for colorectal cancer: a menu of options remains relevant. *Curr Oncol Rep.* 2006;8(6):492-498.
3. O'Leary BA, Olynyk JK, Neville AM, Platell CF. Cost-effectiveness of colorectal cancer screening: comparison of community-based flexible sigmoidoscopy with fecal occult blood testing and colonoscopy. *J Gastroenterol Hepatol.* 2004;19(1):38-47.
4. AGA guideline: colorectal cancer screening and surveillance. *Gastroenterology.* 2003;124:544.
5. Frentz SM, Summers RM. Current status of CT colonography. *Acad Radiol.* 2006;13(12):1517-1531.
6. Cash BD, Schoenfeld P, Rex D. An evidence-based medicine approach to studies of diagnostic tests: assessing the validity of virtual colonoscopy. *Clin Gastroenterol Hepatol.* 2003;1(2):136-144.
7. Powe BD, Finnie R, Ko J. Enhancing knowledge of colorectal cancer among African Americans: why are we waiting until age 50? *Gastroenterol Nurs.* 2006;29(1):42-49.

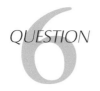
MY PATIENT HAD A 13-MM TUBULAR ADENOMA REMOVED FROM HER COLON. WHAT KIND OF SURVEILLANCE DO I NEED TO RECOMMEND? WOULD IT CHANGE THINGS IF SHE WERE 80 YEARS OLD WITHOUT CO-MORBIDITIES?

Brooks D. Cash, MD, FACP, FACG

Based on current evidence, the answer to the first part of this question can be found in the updated guidelines on colon cancer screening and surveillance put forth by the US Multisociety Task Force on Colorectal Cancer.[1] This document integrates emerging evidence into previously established guidelines and serves as the current roadmap for the primary prevention of colorectal cancer. The patient depicted in the clinical scenario described above fits into the category of people at increased risk for colorectal cancer who should undergo colonoscopic surveillance, and the timing of her next examination should be based on the findings of her previous colonoscopy. Within this category, there is a risk stratification process that needs to occur. Patients with numerous adenomas, a malignant adenoma, a large sessile adenoma, or an incomplete colonoscopy on their previous colonoscopy should undergo a repeat examination within a short time interval. These recommendations do not define several of the parameters involved in making these determinations. At our institution, we define "numerous" adenomas as 10 or more adenomas of any size, a "large" sessile adenoma as ≥1 cm in its longest dimension, and a "short" time interval as 2 to 6 months. According to the guidelines, patients with advanced or multiple (≥3) adenomas should undergo repeat colonoscopy in 3 years.[1] We define an "advanced" adenoma (in accordance with previous trials examining colonoscopy for colorectal cancer screening) as an adenoma that has any of the following characteristics: ≥10 mm in size in any dimension, high-grade dysplasia, or villous histology. The size of our patient's polyp places her into this clinical category, and she should undergo her next colonoscopy in 3 years. Finally, patients found to have 1 to 2 small (<10 mm) adenomas should undergo a repeat colonoscopic screening in 5 to 10 years according to current guidelines.[1] At our institution, we continue to perform surveillance examinations at 5 years for patients in this category.

These recommendations are based on the observations from numerous clinical trials showing that colonoscopic polypectomy and surveillance reduce the incidence of subsequent colorectal cancer by 66% to 90%.[1,2] There is a low annual incidence rate of advanced adenomas and neoplasia after adenomas are removed, and there is randomized controlled trial evidence that the clinical yield of surveillance for patients with a history of advanced adenomas is equivalent at 3 years compared to 1 year.[3] Surveillance examinations accomplish 2 objectives. First, they serve to identify and allow removal of polyps that may have been missed on the first examination. Second, they help to identify patients at risk for interval development of advanced or malignant colorectal polyps. This risk appears to be quite small within the currently recommended surveillance intervals, and it is possible that surveillance examinations are most beneficial for patients with a history of advanced findings on previous colonoscopic examinations. Because of the ability to perform polypectomy during the procedure, colonoscopy is the preferred surveillance examination. The role for less invasive tests for surveillance has not been established but may become appropriate in the future as additional data are accumulated.

The second part of the clinical scenario presented above is more contentious. Current guidelines do not include an age cut-off for colorectal cancer screening or surveillance. While the risk of colorectal cancer increases with age, life expectancy decreases, and this in turn affects the cost-effectiveness of these interventions. There are scant clinical trial data examining the results of colorectal cancer screening or surveillance in the elderly (≥80 years of age) population. One recent trial by Lin and colleagues examined the various types of colorectal neoplasia and compared the mean gain in life expectancy among 1244 patients in 3 age groups (50 to 54 years, 75 to 79 years, ≥80 years) occurring as a result of colorectal cancer screening with colonoscopy.[4] The prevalence of colorectal neoplasia was 13.8% in those 50 to 54 years of age, 26.5% in those 75 to 79 years of age, and 28.6% in those ≥80 years of age. Because the prevalence of advanced neoplasia was higher in the older age groups, these groups benefitted more from screening colonoscopy than the youngest age group. However, when the gains in life expectancy accruing from screening colonoscopy and polypectomy for these groups was calculated, the mean extension in the oldest age group was only 15% of that observed in the youngest age group (0.13 vs 0.85 years). While it is difficult to extrapolate these data to colorectal cancer surveillance, it is reasonable to expect similar outcomes, or perhaps even less benefit, because it is becoming more evident that the primary screening examination is the most crucial factor in terms of reducing the risk of colorectal cancer development in average-risk individuals.

Other studies of colonoscopy in symptomatic and asymptomatic elderly patients have shown that the prevalence of neoplasia in these groups is high. These studies have also shown that cecal intubation rates are lower, procedure times are longer, and perforation rates are higher in very elderly patients. At our institution, we do perform initial colonoscopic screening in patients ≥80 years of age after careful evaluation of their personal wishes, colorectal cancer risk, and medical comorbidities. We also apply these policies to patients presenting for surveillance examinations. Beyond age 80, if the previous colonoscopy did not reveal any advanced neoplasia, we typically recommend no further examinations. If the previous colonoscopy did reveal advanced neoplasia and there are no major medical co-morbidities, we will typically recommend a surveillance examination based upon the previously discussed surveillance guidelines. It is important to realize that screening and surveillance in such patients need to be individualized and carefully implemented with appropriate counseling and that, at the current time, there is no all-inclusive "right" answer to the second part of the clinical scenario presented above.

References

1. Winawer SJ, Zauber AG, Fletcher RH, et al. Guidelines for colonoscopy surveillance after polypectomy: a consensus update by the US Multi-Society Task Force on Colorectal Cancer and the American Cancer Society. *CA Cancer J Clin.* 2006;56(3):143-159.
2. Singh H, Turner D, Xue L, Targownik LE, Bernstein CN. Risk of developing colorectal cancer following a negative colonoscopy examination: evidence for a 10-year interval between colonoscopies. *JAMA.* 2006;295(20):2366-2373.
3. Pabby A, Schoen RE, Weissfeld JL, et al. Analysis of colorectal cancer occurrence during surveillance colonoscopy in the dietary Polyp Prevention Trial. *Gastrointest Endosc.* 2005;61(3):385-391.
4. Lin OS, Kozarek RA, Schembre DB, et al. Screening colonoscopy in very elderly patients: prevalence of neoplasia and estimated impact on life expectancy. *JAMA.* 2006;295(20):2357-2365.

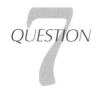

I HAVE A PATIENT WHOSE BROTHER, MOTHER, AND MATERNAL UNCLE ALL HAD COLON CANCER DIAGNOSED BEFORE THE AGE OF 45. DOES MY PATIENT HAVE HEREDITARY NONPOLYPOSIS COLORECTAL CANCER SYNDROME, AND, IF HE DOES, WHAT SHOULD I ADVISE?

Brooks D. Cash, MD, FACP, FACG

Hereditary nonpolyposis colorectal cancer (HNPCC), also known as Lynch syndrome, is a dominantly inherited colorectal cancer syndrome that is responsible for approximately 5% of the yearly colorectal cancer burden and is estimated to affect between 1/1000 and 1/2000 individuals. HNPCC is associated with early-onset cancers in the gastrointestinal tract and other parts of the body including the uterus, urologic tract, ovaries, and brain.[1] Genetic mutations can be found in the majority of families with HNPCC, and genetic testing is an important adjunct in the clinical care and counseling of kindreds with HNPCC. Aggressive screening for colorectal cancer has been shown to decrease the incidence, stage, and mortality of colorectal disease associated with HNPCC.

The lifetime risk of colorectal cancer in HNPCC is thought to be approximately 80%, with a mean age of onset of 44 years. Most of the tumors (70%) are right sided (proximal to the splenic flexure) and carry a high risk of metachronous colorectal cancer at 10 years. The histologic characteristics of HNPCC-associated colorectal cancers can alert the astute clinician to the possibility of the syndrome. These features include mucinous/signet ring cell or poorly differentiated cancers, particularly when accompanied by tumor-infiltrating lymphocytes (TIL) in non-mucinous or poorly differentiated cancers or a lymphoid response similar to that seen in Crohn's disease. In women with HNPCC, the risk of developing endometrial cancers is even greater than that of colorectal cancer, and more than 50% of these women will present with gynecologic cancers as their first malignancy at a mean age of 44 years.[2]

HNPCC arises due to a germline mutation in one of several DNA mismatch repair (MMR) genes. Identified mutation targets include MSH2, MLH1, MSH6, and PMS2. The presence of one of these mutations is considered the "first hit." When another acquired genetic alteration or loss of the other allele occurs, tumor suppression is compromised and carcinogenesis occurs. With accumulating MMR mutations, the host is unable to repair damage to the ubiquitous DNA replication errors in tumor cells and short, repeated sequences of DNA known as microsatellites are produced. Microsatellite instability (MSI) is the molecular fingerprint of HNPCC-related tumors and can be found in up to 90% of tumors from individuals who fulfill the Amsterdam criteria for HNPCC.

Most HNPCC kindreds will be identified through a careful history. The Amsterdam criteria depend on using pedigree as well as information regarding the age of onset, location, and pathology of tumors in order to identify potential HNPCC kindreds and are highly specific.[1] These criteria require (1) three relatives with colorectal cancer, (2) two successive generations affected, (3) one of the relatives must be a first-degree relative with the other two, (4) the onset of cancer in at least 1 relative at age <50 years, and (5) familial adenomatous polyposis (FAP), another familial colorectal cancer syndrome characterized by hundreds of colonic adenomas and specific phenotypic abnormalities, should also be excluded.

The newer Amsterdam II criteria incorporate extracolonic tumors into the decision matrix and should be considered when a prolific family history of cancer, especially at age <50 years, is uncovered during the review of patient history.[3] Based on the clinical scenario and criteria above, we should be concerned that our patient does belong to a HNPCC kindred.

In the current scenario, it certainly appears that our patient fulfills the Amsterdam criteria. The patient should be referred for colonoscopic evaluation. For patients known to have HNPCC, colonoscopic screening should occur every 1 to 3 years beginning at age 20 to 25, or 10 to 15 years younger than the age at diagnosis of the youngest person diagnosed with cancer in the family.[4] Colonoscopic surveillance at these intervals has been shown to reduce the incidence and stage of colorectal cancer by 40% to 60% and has also been shown to reduce colorectal cancer mortality in one study from the Netherlands. For women, annual gynecologic surveillance should begin at age 25 to 35 with transvaginal ultrasonography, CA-125, and endometrial aspiration. For individuals from kindreds with a history of urologic or gastric cancers, annual urine cytology and gastroscopy every 1 to 2 years beginning at age 30 to 35 is recommended by some experts.

If the presence of HNPCC is not known, the evaluation becomes more complicated. If possible, the resected tumors of family members should undergo testing for MSI or immunohistochemical staining to identify the loss of protein products from affected MMR genes. Commercially available genetic tests are also available, but are costly and controversial. Their ability to detect mutations is variable, ranging from 40% to 77%, and individuals should be carefully considered and counseled before undergoing such testing. Ideally, genetic testing should be performed in an individual who is affected with the disease.[5] If a mutation is found, then other family members should be offered genetic testing to more accurately predict their risk. If no mutations are found, then the at-risk status of family members cannot be determined, and they should continue to undergo aggressive surveillance.

When there are no family members available to test, there are some clinical prediction rules available that may help determine who would be most likely to benefit from genetic testing. One of these is from the Dana-Farber Cancer Institute and is known as the PREMM1,2 model. It is available online at http://www.dfci.org/pat/cancer/gastrointestinal/crc-calculator/default.asp. If the Predicted Probability of Mutation is more than 5%, the individual should be considered for a genetic evaluation. If such an evaluation is to be carried out, it is highly recommended that the patient be sent to a center that specializes in the care of individuals with HNPCC and their families because such evaluations can have wide-ranging ramifications.

References

1. Vasen HF, Mecklin JP, Khan PM, Lynch HT. The international collaborative group on hereditary non-polyposis colorectal cancer (ICG-HNPCC). *Dis Colon Rectum.* 1991;34(5):424-425.
2. Ericson K, Nilbert M, Bladstrom A, et al. Familial risk of tumors associated with hereditary nonpolyposis colorectal cancer: a Swedish population based study. *Scand J Gastroenterol.* 2004;39(12):1259-1265.
3. Lynch HT, de la Chapelle A. Hereditary colorectal cancer. *N Engl J Med.* 2003;348(10):919-932.
4. Winawer SJ, Fletcher R, Rex D. Colorectal cancer screening and surveillance: clinical guidelines and rationale. Update based on new evidence. *Gastroenterology.* 2003;124(2):544-560.
5. Burke W, Petersen G, Lynch P, et al. Recommendations for follow-up care of individuals with an inherited predisposition to cancer: I. Hereditary nonpolyposis colon cancer. *JAMA.* 1997;277(11):915-919.

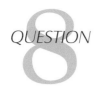
WHAT DO I NEED TO TELL MY INFLAMMATORY BOWEL DISEASE PATIENTS ABOUT THEIR RISK FOR COLON CANCER AND HOW SHOULD I PERFORM SURVEILLANCE COLONOSCOPY IN THESE PATIENTS?

Francis A. Farraye, MD, MSc

Patients with long-standing ulcerative colitis are at an increased risk for developing dysplasia and CRC. This risk approaches 8% by 20 years and 18% by 30 years.[1] More recent data suggest that the risk of CRC in patients with ulcerative colitis may be lower than previously reported.[2] Patients with extensive Crohn's colitis also have an increased risk of CRC and should undergo regular surveillance.

A number of factors are associated with an increased risk of developing CRC in inflammatory bowel disease (IBD). These include a longer duration of colitis, greater extent of colonic involvement, family history of CRC, primary sclerosing cholangitis (PSC), young age of IBD onset, and possibly backwash ileitis. A number of factors may lower the risk of developing dysplasia and/or CRC. These include prophylactic total proctocolectomy, surveillance programs to detect dysplasia or early-stage asymptomatic CRC, and possibly chemoprevention with 5-ASAs, folate, ursodiol, and NSAIDs.

At present, despite a lack of evidence from randomized controlled trials, surveillance colonoscopy is the best and most widely used method to detect dysplasia and cancer in patients with IBD (Table 8-1).[3-5] It is recommended that all ulcerative colitis patients undergo colonoscopy with biopsies throughout the colon approximately 8 years after the onset of symptoms to determine the endoscopic and microscopic extent of colitis. It is also

---

Table 8-1
Suggested Performance of Surveillance Colonoscopy

- Beginning approximately 7 to 8 years from the onset of colitis, all patients with ulcerative colitis should undergo an initial screening colonoscopy to determine the extent of colitis and check for neoplasia.
- Patients with left-sided colitis should follow the same schedule as those with extensive colitis, although some authorities suggest that regular surveillance for left-sided colitis should begin after 15 years of disease when the risk rises to that of extensive colitis.
- In the case of patients with primary sclerosing cholangitis, screening colonoscopy should be carried out at the time the biliary tract disease is diagnosed.
- If no dysplasia is detected, patients with extensive colitis (proximal to the hepatic flexure) should have repeat examinations every 1 to 2 years.
- If indefinite dysplasia is reported, the nature of the uncertainty should be ascertained from the pathologist. If the suspicion of dysplasia is high (ie, probably positive), short-term rebiopsy within 3 to 6 months or less may be indicated; if low (ie, probably negative), the interval should be reduced to every 6 to 12 months.
- Obtain 4 biopsy specimens of flat mucosa every 10 cm (consider sampling every 5 cm in the rectosigmoid).
- Place each quadruplicate set in a separate specimen jar (as opposed to pooling biopsy specimens from several colonic segments).
- Sample suspicious lesions or polyps.
- Make sure to biopsy flat mucosa around the base of any suspicious polyp and submit specimen in a separate container.
- Consider suppressing symptoms of active inflammation with medical therapy prior to surveillance colonoscopy.
- In Crohn's colitis, strictures may require using a thinner caliber colonoscope.
- Consider brush cytology or barium enema to evaluate impassable strictures.

Adapted with permission from Itzkowitz SH, Harpaz N. Diagnosis and management of dysplasia in patients with inflammatory bowel diseases. *Gastroenterology.* 2004;126(6):1634-1648.

---

generally accepted that patients with extensive Crohn's colitis, defined by involvement of at least one-third of the colon, should undergo surveillance colonoscopy. Patients with IBD and PSC should have yearly colonoscopies once the diagnosis of PSC is established. In patients with pan-colitis, at least 33 random biopsies should be taken throughout the colon with more biopsies in the rectum and sigmoid as several studies suggest that dysplasia is more common in these areas. I take 6 biopsies per pathology specimen bottle taken from the right colon, transverse colon, descending colon, sigmoid colon, and proximal and distal rectum in patients with pan-colitis. Suspicious polypoid lesions should be removed by snare cautery. Additional biopsies should be taken from around the lesion and placed in a separate container. If no dysplasia is identified, colonoscopy should be performed every 1 to 3 years until 20 years of disease, and then every 1 to 2 years thereafter, although recommendations regarding intervals vary.

There are several limitations to surveillance colonoscopy, and colonoscopy practices are not uniform. Obtaining multiple biopsies is time consuming, and there are only moderate levels of agreement among pathologists on the diagnosis of dysplasia. Colonoscopic biopsies

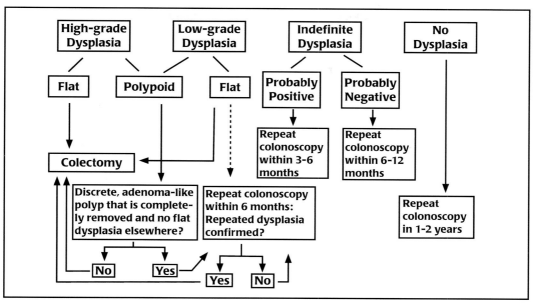

Figure 8-1. Suggested surveillance strategy for patients with IBD. (Reproduced with permission from Itzkowitz SH, Harpaz N. Diagnosis and management of dysplasia in patients with inflammatory bowel diseases. *Gastroenterology.* 2004;126[6]:1634-1648.)

should be characterized pathologically as negative; indefinite for dysplasia; or positive for low-grade dysplasia (LGD), high-grade dysplasia (HGD) or carcinoma, and an expert GI pathologist should confirm all cases of dysplasia. Patients with ulcerative proctitis or ulcerative proctosigmoiditis do not have an increased risk of developing colorectal cancer and do not need to be in an intensive surveillance program, but rather follow average-risk CRC screening guidelines.

The finding of flat HGD confirmed by two expert GI pathologists or carcinoma in endoscopic biopsy samples is an indication for colectomy. There is accumulating evidence to suggest that flat LGD is also an indication for colectomy because of the relatively high rate of progression to HGD or cancer.[6] Blackstone and colleagues first described the term dysplasia associated lesion or mass (DALM) in 1981. In Blackstone's study of 12 patients with DALMs, 7 were malignant and consequently any raised dysplastic lesion was felt to be an indication for colectomy.[7] However, it is now apparent that DALMs actually represent a heterogeneous population of tumors in which the cancer risk is not equal. Raised dysplastic lesions with the appearance of sporadic adenomas have been termed adenoma-like DALMs, and recent studies have demonstrated that patients with adenoma-like DALMs, with either low-grade or high-grade dysplasia, may be treated adequately by polypectomy and continued surveillance.[8-10] Non-adenoma-like DALMs still remain an indication for colectomy because of their high association with CRC. Close follow-up endoscopic surveillance is required for patients in whom a polypoid dysplastic lesion is removed (Figure 8-1).

Given the inherent difficulties in the performance of surveillance colonoscopy, it has been suggested that chemoprevention be explored as a method to lower the risk of developing dysplasia and CRC in IBD. Chemoprevention refers to the use of drugs to reverse, suppress, or delay the process of carcinogenesis. Several agents have been suggested as chemopreventive agents including folic acid, ursodeoxycholic acid, NSAIDs and 5-ASAs. A discussion of chemoprevention is beyond the scope of this presentation but the reader is referred to a recent review for additional information.[11] It must be made clear that there is insufficient evidence to modify present screening and surveillance practices in IBD patients on these medications and that chemoprevention is not a substitute for surveillance colonoscopy.

In summary, patients with long-standing ulcerative colitis and extensive Crohn's colitis are at an increased risk for developing CRC. The finding of flat HGD confirmed by an expert GI pathologist is an indication for colectomy in a patient with IBD. Although somewhat controversial, accumulating evidence suggests that flat LGD is also an indication for colectomy. If colectomy is not performed for flat LGD or HGD, then close follow-up with repeat colonoscopy (3 months) with multiple biopsies is warranted. Polypoid dysplasia that is completely excised and unassociated with flat dysplasia surrounding the polyp or elsewhere in the colon can be managed by polypectomy alone and continued colonoscopic surveillance.

References

1. Eaden J. Review article: colorectal carcinoma and inflammatory bowel disease. *Aliment Pharmacol Ther.* 2004;20 (suppl 4):24-30.
2. Loftus EV Jr. Epidemiology and risk factors for colorectal dysplasia and cancer in ulcerative colitis. *Gastroenterol Clin North Am.* 2006;35(3):517-531.
3. Eaden JA, Mayberry JF. Guidelines for screening and surveillance of asymptomatic colorectal cancer in patients with inflammatory bowel disease. *Gut.* 2002;51 (suppl 5):V10-12.
4. Itzkowitz SH, Harpaz N. Diagnosis and management of dysplasia in patients with inflammatory bowel diseases. *Gastroenterology.* 2004;126(6):1634-1648.
5. Itzkowitz SH, Present DH. Consensus conference: colorectal cancer screening and surveillance in inflammatory bowel disease. *Inflamm Bowel Dis.* 2005;11(3):314-321.
6. Ullman T, Croog V, Harpaz N, et al. Progression of flat low-grade dysplasia to advanced neoplasia in patients with ulcerative colitis. *Gastroenterology.* 2003;125(5):1311-1319.
7. Blackstone MO, Riddell RH, Rogers BH, Levin B. Dysplasia-associated lesion or mass (DALM) detected by colonoscopy in long-standing ulcerative colitis: an indication for colectomy. *Gastroenterology.* 1981;80(2):366-374.
8. Friedman S, Odze RD, Farraye FA. Management of neoplastic polyps in inflammatory bowel disease. *Inflamm Bowel Dis.* 2003;9(4):260-266.
9. Odze RD, Farraye FA, Hecht JL, Hornick JL. Long-term follow-up after polypectomy treatment for adenoma-like dysplastic lesions in ulcerative colitis. *Clin Gastroenterol Hepatol.* 2004;2(7):534-541.
10. Rubin PH, Friedman S, Harpaz N, et al. Colonoscopic polypectomy in chronic colitis: conservative management after endoscopic resection of dysplastic polyps. *Gastroenterology.* 1999;117(6):1295-1300.
11. Chan EP, Lichtenstein GR. Chemoprevention: risk reduction with medical therapy of inflammatory bowel disease. *Gastroenterol Clin North Am.* 2006;35(3):675-712.

WHAT DO I TELL THE SURGEONS WHO INSIST ON ANNUAL COLONOSCOPIES FOR PATIENTS WITH CURED COLON CANCER, EVEN FOR THOSE 5 TO 10 YEARS PAST THERAPY?

Brooks D. Cash, MD, FACP, FACG

Recommendations on the use of surveillance colonoscopy after resection of colorectal cancer were recently produced jointly by the US Multi-Society Task Force on Colorectal Cancer and the American Cancer Society (ACS).[1] They constitute the updated recommendations of both organizations. These guidelines were endorsed by the Colorectal Cancer Advisory Committee of the ACS and by the governing boards of the American College of Gastroenterology, the American Gastroenterological Association, and the American Society for Gastrointestinal Endoscopy and represent the most up-to-date evidence-based recommendations for the surveillance of patients with a history of colorectal cancer (Tables 9-1 and 9-2).

In general, patients who undergo surgical resection of Stage I, II, or III colon and rectal cancers, or curative-intent resection of Stage IV cancers are candidates for surveillance colonoscopy. Patients who undergo curative endoscopic resection of Stage I colon cancers are also candidates for surveillance colonoscopy. Patients with Stage IV colon or rectal cancer that is unresectable for cure are generally not candidates for surveillance colonoscopy because their chance of survival from their primary cancer is low, and the risks of surveillance outweigh any potential benefit.[2]

It is important to realize that historically there have been two primary goals for surveillance of patients with a history of resected colorectal cancer that have prompted clinicians to perform frequent surveillance procedures. The first is the detection of early recurrence of the primary tumor at a stage that will permit curative treatment. The sec-

---

Table 9-1

Current Postcancer Resection Surveillance Guidelines

- Patients with colon and rectal cancer should undergo high-quality perioperative clearing. In the case of nonobstructing tumors, this can be done by preoperative colonoscopy. In the case of obstructing colon cancers, computed tomography colonography with intravenous contrast or double contrast barium enema can be used to detect neoplasms in the proximal colon. In these cases, a colonoscopy to clear the colon of synchronous disease should be considered 3 to 6 months after the resection if no unresectable metastases are found during surgery. Alternatively, colonoscopy can be performed intraoperatively.
- Patients undergoing curative resection for colon or rectal cancer should undergo a colonoscopy 1 year after the resection (or 1 year after the performance of the colonoscopy that was performed to clear the colon of synchronous disease). This colonoscopy at 1 year is in addition to the perioperative colonoscopy for synchronous tumors.
- If the examination performed at 1 year is normal, then the interval before the next subsequent examination should be 3 years. If that colonoscopy is normal, then the interval before the next subsequent examination should be 5 years.
- Following the examination at 1 year, the intervals before subsequent examinations may be shortened if there is evidence of hereditary nonpolyposis colorectal cancer or if adenoma findings warrant earlier colonoscopy.
- Periodic examination of the rectum for the purpose of identifying local recurrence, usually performed at 3- to 6-month intervals for the first 2 or 3 years, may be considered after low anterior resection of rectal cancer. The techniques utilized are typically rigid proctoscopy, flexible proctoscopy, or rectal endoscopic ultrasound. These examinations are independent of the colonoscopic examinations described above for detection of metachronous disease.

---

ond goal is to search for and identify metachronous colorectal cancers. In regard to detection of recurrences of the initial primary cancer, serial measurements of carcinoembryonic antigen are widely used. In addition, recent meta-analyses of randomized controlled trials suggest that annual chest x-rays and computed tomography (CT) scans of the liver can improve survival from the original primary cancer by early detection of surgically curable recurrences.[3]

The answer to the question posed is simply that neither individual randomized controlled trials of intensive surveillance with colonoscopy, nor meta-analyses of these trials, have demonstrated a survival benefit from the original primary tumor by performing colonoscopy at annual or shorter intervals.[3,4] The rationale that yearly colonoscopy for patients with resected colorectal cancer will identify anastomotic or intraluminal recurrences that are amenable to curative therapy has simply not been borne out to be true. Several studies have shown that the low rate of these recurrences after resection do not merit surveillance colonoscopy and that even when such an unfortunate event occurs, the disease is usually already extended into the abdomen or pelvis and can rarely be resected for cure.[5] Thus, the performance of annual colonoscopy for the purpose of detecting recurrent disease does not have an established survival benefit for patients with colorectal cancer. The more immediate goal of surveillance is to detect metachronous cancers.

An exception to the above occurs in the case of rectal cancer. In contrast to the anastomotic recurrence rate of 2% to 4% seen with colon cancer, the rate of anastomotic recur-

> ## Table 9-2
> # Additional Postcancer Surveillance Recommendations
>
> - An acceptable colonoscopy is complete to the cecum, and bowel preparation is adequate.
> - A continuous quality improvement process is critical to the effective application of colonoscopy in colorectal cancer prevention.
> - Endoscopists should make clear recommendations to primary care physicians about when the next colonoscopy is indicated.
> - Performance of fecal occult blood test is discouraged in patients undergoing colonoscopic surveillance.
> - Discontinuation of surveillance colonoscopy should be considered in people with advanced age or comorbidities (with <10 years of life expectancy), according to the clinician's judgment.
> - Surveillance guidelines are intended for asymptomatic people. New symptoms may need diagnostic workup.
> - Chromoendoscopy (dye-spraying) and magnification endoscopy are not established as essential to screening or surveillance.
> - Computed tomography colonography (virtual colonoscopy) is not established as a surveillance modality.

rence in rectal cancer may be 10 times higher. High recurrence rates of rectal cancer are partly a function of surgical technique and volume. Specifically, recurrence rates below 10% have been consistently reported when patients are operated on by a technique called total mesorectal excision.[6] This technique involves sharp dissection of the rectum and its surrounding adventitia along the first plane outside the adventitia (the mesorectal fascia). Local recurrence rates of rectal cancer can be further reduced by administration of chemotherapy and radiation therapy, which have been most effectively administered in the neoadjuvant (preoperative) setting to patients with locally advanced disease. Therefore, knowledge of surgical technique and other therapies is important to ascertain when considering surveillance of patients with a history of rectal cancer. Because local recurrence rates for rectal cancer across the United States are generally higher than those achieved in series utilizing total mesorectal excision, there is a rationale for performing periodic examinations of the rectum by rigid or flexible proctoscopy or endoscopic ultrasound. Current recommendations include periodic examination of the rectum for the purpose of identifying local recurrence, usually performed at 3- to 6-month intervals for the first 2 or 3 years after low anterior resection of rectal cancer. These techniques have not been shown to improve survival, and the only rationale for their use is high rates of local recurrence.

With regard to metachronous cancers, among 23 studies in which patients underwent perioperative clearing by colonoscopy, 157 colonoscopies were required per metachronous cancer detected, which compares favorably to the rate of prevalent cancers detected during screening colonoscopy of approximately 135.[5] Among studies of postcancer resection surveillance colonoscopy, there were 57 metachronous cancers in the first 2 years after resection of the initial primary, with an incidence rate of 0.7% over this interval. Nearly two-thirds of these metachronous cancers were Dukes' Stage A or B, slightly more than half were asymptomatic, and nearly 90% of patients in these studies underwent opera-

Figure 9-1. Recurrent adenocarcinoma found at 1-year surveillance colonoscopy after curative resection of colorectal cancer. This mass was located 3 cm distal to the colo-colonic anastamosis in the descending colon.

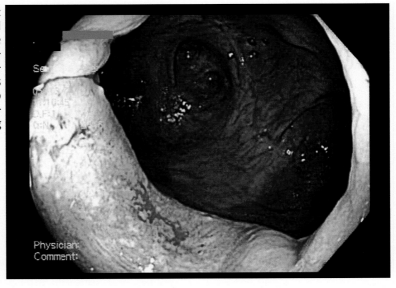

tions with curative intent. Taken together, these findings were considered sufficient to warrant a colonoscopy 1 year after resection or after the perioperative clearing colonoscopy for the purpose of identification of apparently metachronous colorectal neoplasms (Figure 9-1). The recommendation to perform a colonoscopy at 1 year does not diminish the need for high quality in the performance of the perioperative clearing examination for synchronous neoplasms. If the examination performed at 1 year is normal, then the interval before the next subsequent examination should be 3 years.[1] If that colonoscopy is normal, then the interval before the next subsequent examination should be every 5 years. Shorter intervals should be reserved for patients whose age, family history, or tumor testing indicate definite or probable hereditary nonpolyposis colorectal cancer. This is what should be communicated to your colleagues who insist on annual surveillance examinations 3 to 5 years after curative resection of the primary colon cancer.

References

1. Rex DK, Kahi CJ, Levin B, et al. Guidelines for colonoscopy surveillance after cancer resection: a consensus update by the American Cancer Society and US Multi-Society Task Force on Colorectal Cancer. *CA Cancer J Clin.* 2006;56(3):160-167.
2. Pagana TJ, Ledesma EJ, Mittelman A, et al. The use of colonoscopy in the study of synchronous colorectal neoplasms. *Cancer.* 1984;53(2):356-359.
3. Jeffery GM, Hickey BE, Hider P. Follow-up strategies for patients treated for nonmetastatic colorectal cancer. *Cochrane Database Syst Rev.* 2002;(1):CD002200.
4. Renehan AG, Egger M, Saunders MP, et al. Impact on survival of intensive follow up after curative resection for colorectal cancer: systematic review and meta-analysis of randomised trials. *BMJ.* 2002;324(7341):813.
5. Cali RL, Pitsch RM, Thorson AG, et al. Cumulative incidence of metachronous colorectal cancer. *Dis Colon Rectum.* 1993;36(4):388-393.
6. Kapiteijn E, Marijnen CA, Nagtegaal ID, et al. Dutch Colorectal Cancer Group. Preoperative radiotherapy combined with total mesorectal excision for resectable rectal cancer. *N Engl J Med.* 2001;345(9):638-646.

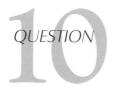

QUESTION

10

THE PATHOLOGISTS KEEP SENDING ME REPORTS ABOUT SERRATED ADENOMAS. WHAT IS A SERRATED ADENOMA AND WHAT DO I TELL MY PATIENTS IN TERMS OF FOLLOW-UP?

Christopher S. Huang, MD
Francis A. Farraye, MD, MSc
Michael J. O'Brien, MD, MPH

Serrated adenomas are polyps that simultaneously demonstrate the serrated architecture typical of hyperplastic polyps and the epithelial dysplasia of conventional adenomas.[1] They are a subset of a larger group of polyps collectively known as serrated polyps, which are characterized by the histologic feature of "saw-toothed" (serrated) infolding of the crypt epithelium. Hyperplastic polyps (HPs) are the most common type of serrated polyp and have long been regarded as completely innocuous lesions with no malignant potential. While this viewpoint is valid for the majority of small HPs, particularly in the distal colon, we now recognize that some HPs represent precursor lesions in an alternative pathway to colon cancer, termed the serrated pathway.[2,3] Although its actual contribution to the overall burden of colon cancer is not precisely known, it has been estimated that the serrated pathway accounts for up to 10% to 15% of all colon cancers, and represents the primary pathway to sporadic cancers with microsatellite instability (MSI).[4] Thus, serrated adenomas and other serrated polyps have recently received a great deal of attention.

There are several types of serrated polyps, which can be classified based on the presence or absence of dysplasia (Table 10-1). Non-dysplastic serrated polyps include the lesions commonly known as HPs (of which there are actually several subtypes) and an atypical HP variant known as the sessile serrated adenoma (SSA), sessile serrated polyp (SSP), or serrated polyp with abnormal proliferation (SPAP). Unfortunately, this nomen-

---

Table 10-1

Classification of Serrated Polyps

Non-dysplastic Serrated Lesions	*Dysplastic Serrated Lesions*
Aberrant crypt foci, hyperplastic type	Serrated adenoma
Hyperplastic polyp	Admixed polyp (a dysplastic serrated
Microvesicular serrated polyp	polyp that contains a non-dysplastic
Goblet cell serrated polyp	serrated component and a non-ser-
Mucin depleted serrated polyp	rated dysplastic component resembling
Sessile serrated adenoma (sessile serrat-	a conventional adenoma)
ed polyp, serrated polyp with abnormal	Serrated adenocarcinoma
proliferation)	

---

clature is confusing and, it must be emphasized, despite its "adenoma" designation, the SSA is non-dysplastic and is a distinct entity from the serrated adenoma, a dysplastic serrated polyp. The relationships between the various serrated polyps are still being defined, but molecular genetic studies have linked a HP subtype known as the microvesicular serrated polyp with SSAs, serrated adenomas, and serrated cancers, based on their high concordance of BRAF mutations and CpG island methylation status.[5,6] The progression of nondysplastic serrated polyps to dysplastic serrated polyps and ultimately to serrated cancers is associated with increasing levels of CpG island methylation, which results in inactivation of important tumor-suppressor and mutator genes (eg, hMLH1, a DNA mismatch repair gene). High levels of MSI frequently characterize the cancers that arise as an endpoint of this pathway. A second, less well-defined arm of the serrated pathway is associated with KRAS (as opposed to BRAF) mutation, low levels of CpG island methylation, and endpoint cancers that are microsatellite stable, sharing features similar to those of APC-mutated cancers of the conventional adenoma-carcinoma sequence. The postulated pathways are illustrated in Figure 10-1.

Serrated adenomas (Figure 10-2) are actually quite uncommon, compared to conventional adenomas, SSAs, and HPs. In the original report describing this entity, serrated adenomas represented only 101 of more than 18,000 polyps reviewed (<0.6%).[1] In contrast to SSAs, which occur predominantly in the proximal colon, serrated adenomas are more prevalent distally. They may be flat, sessile, or polypoid and may show a tubular, tubulovillous, or villous architecture. In one study of 357 serrated adenomas, 240 (67%) were polypoid and 127 (33%) were superficial (sessile or flat). The superficial serrated adenomas had a significantly larger diameter than polypoid serrated adenomas (mean 10.1 mm vs 6.3 mm) and were more commonly located in the proximal colon, reflecting their likely origin in SSAs. A tubulovillous growth pattern was common in polypoid serrated adenomas (31.5%).[7]

Despite their rarity, serrated adenomas are nonetheless important because of their malignant potential. The magnitude of cancer risk in patients with serrated adenomas is not known. Studies have reported a prevalence rate of high-grade dysplasia and intramu-

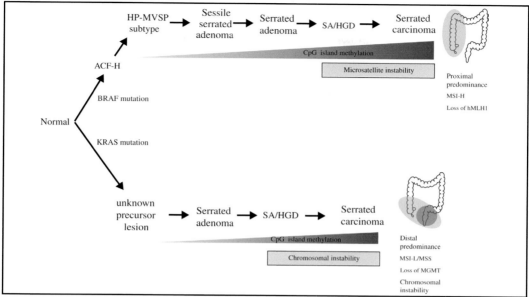

Figure 10-1. Schematic illustration of the postulated serrated pathways to colon cancer. ACF-H = aberrant crypt foci-hyperplastic type; HP = hyperplastic polyp; MVSP = microvesicular serrated polyp; SA/HGD = serrated adenoma with high-grade dysplasia.

cosal carcinoma within serrated adenomas ranging from 5% to 37% and 4% to 11%, respectively.[1,8-13] It is likely that the risk of malignant progression varies significantly with the size and location of the serrated adenoma, as suggested by one study in which 1.5% of serrated adenomas smaller than 10 mm demonstrated concomitant carcinoma, compared to 10% of those 10 mm or larger.[13] Serrated adenomas that arise from precursor SSAs may share the aggressive nature of adenomas in patients with hereditary nonpolyposis colon cancer syndrome (HNPCC), related to defective DNA mismatch repair and high levels of MSI (MSI-H). Several studies have indicated, however, that MSI-H develops late in serrated adenomas and is concordant with the appearance of high-grade dysplasia or carcinoma. It is clear that serrated adenomas are premalignant lesions that should be treated with at least the same degree of diligence as that afforded conventional advanced adenomas in terms of resection and postpolypectomy surveillance. Therefore, we currently recommend surveillance colonoscopy in 3 to 5 years after complete resection of a serrated adenoma.

A greater dilemma revolves around the management of SSAs. The first challenge is to recognize the lesion (Figure 10-3)—SSAs are typically subtle, smooth lesions, frequently covered with mucus, show poor endoscopic circumscription (often having the appearance of a prominent fold of mucosa), and are encountered mainly in the proximal colon. These endoscopic features should prompt the endoscopist to attempt complete resection whenever possible and to specifically ask the pathologist whether the lesion represents an SSA. In contrast to serrated adenomas, SSAs are quite common, representing 9% of all polyps in a recent study of consecutive patients in whom high-resolution chromoendoscopy was performed in the proximal colon.[14] Unfortunately, there are limited data to guide the clinical management of these growth-disordered but non-dysplastic lesions. Until more

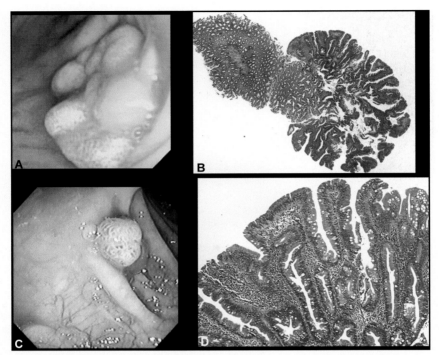

Figure 10-2. Endoscopic appearance and histology of serrated adenoma. (A) A serrated adenoma of the proximal colon that shows smooth and cerebriform surface patterns with a sessile shape. (B) Histology of Figure A, showing a dysplastic serrated polyp (serrated adenoma) at right, contiguous with non-dysplastic serrated polyp precursor classified as sessile serrated adenoma. (C) A pedunculated serrated adenoma of the descending colon. (D) Histology of Figure C showing a polyp with serration and dysplasia. Huang CS, O'Brien MJ, Yang S, Farraye FA. Hyperplastic polyps, serrated adenomas, and the serrated polyp neoplasia pathway. (Reprinted with permission from Huang CS, O'Brien MJ, Yang S, Farraye FA. Hyperplastic polyps, serrated adenomas, and the serrated polyp neoplasia pathway. *Am J Gastroenterol.* 2004;99[11]:2242-2255.)

is known, we feel it is prudent to assign a single SSA the same status of a small tubular adenoma and recommend complete resection followed by surveillance colonoscopy 5 years after resection.

Finally, although evidence is accumulating to support the potential for neoplastic progression of some HPs, we acknowledge that it is impractical and unnecessary to advocate removal of every single minute HP, especially those located in the distal colon and rectum. However, certain clinical and endoscopic features may identify HPs that warrant special consideration, such as multiplicity (>20), large size (>10 mm), proximal location, and positive family history of colon cancer.[15] These features may point to underlying hyperplastic polyposis syndrome or identify patients at risk for developing cancer via the serrated pathway.

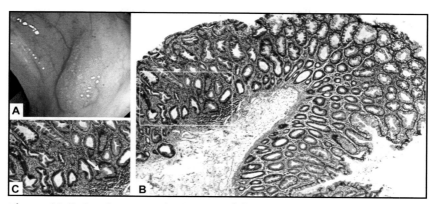

Figure 10-3. Sessile serrated adenoma. (A) Mucus-covered sessile polyp on the crest of a mucosal fold. (B) Histological section shows a sessile serrated adenoma (atypical hyperplastic polyp). This serrated polyp overall resembles a hyperplastic polyp (microvesicular variant) but an area of the polyp (C inset) shows disordered growth patterns in the crypt bases represented by irregular branching (green arrow), long axes parallel to the surface, and goblet cells in the crypt base (white arrow).

References

1. Longacre TA, Fenoglio-Preiser CM. Mixed hyperplastic adenomatous polyps/serrated adenomas. A distinct form of colorectal neoplasia. *Am J Surg Pathol.* 1990;14(6):524-537.
2. Jass JR, Whitehall VL, Young J, Leggett BA. Emerging concepts in colorectal neoplasia. *Gastroenterology.* 2002;123(3):862-876.
3. Huang CS, O'Brien MJ, Yang S, Farraye FA. Hyperplastic polyps, serrated adenomas, and the serrated polyp neoplasia pathway. *Am J Gastroenterol.* 2004;99(11):2242-2255.
4. Makinen MJ. Colorectal serrated adenocarcinoma. *Histopathology.* 2007;50(1):131-150.
5. O'Brien MJ, Yang S, Mack C, et al. Comparison of microsatellite instability, CpG island methylation phenotype, BRAF and KRAS status in serrated polyps and traditional adenomas indicates separate pathways to distinct colorectal carcinoma end points. *Am J Surg Pathol.* 2006;30(12):1491-1501.
6. O'Brien MJ. Hyperplastic and serrated polyps of the colorectum. *Gastroenterol Clin North Am.* 2007;36(4):947-968.
7. Oka S, Tanaka S, Hiyama T, et al. Clinicopathologic and endoscopic features of colorectal serrated adenoma: differences between polypoid and superficial types. *Gastrointest Endosc.* 2004;59(2):213-219.
8. Jaramillo E, Watanabe M, Rubio C, Slezak P. Small colorectal serrated adenomas: endoscopic findings. *Endoscopy.* 1997;29(1):1-3.
9. Matsumoto T, Mizuno M, Shimizu M, Manabe T, Iida M. Clinicopathological features of serrated adenoma of the colorectum: comparison with traditional adenoma. *J Clin Pathol.* 1999;52(7):513-516.
10. Matsumoto T, Mizuno M, Shimizu M, et al. Serrated adenoma of the colorectum: colonoscopic and histologic features. *Gastrointest Endosc.* 1999;49(6):736-742.
11. Yao T, Kouzuki T, Kajiwara M, et al. "Serrated" adenoma of the colorectum, with reference to its gastric differentiation and its malignant potential. *J Pathol.* 1999;187(5):511-517.
12. Rubio CA, Jaramillo E. Flat serrated adenomas of the colorectal mucosa. *Jpn J Cancer Res.* 1996;87(3):305-309.
13. Iwabuchi M, Sasano H, Hiwatashi N, et al. Serrated adenoma: a clinicopathological, DNA ploidy, and immunohistochemical study. *Anticancer Res.* 2000;20(2B):1141-1147.
14. Spring KJ, Zhao ZZ, Karamatic R, et al. High prevalence of sessile serrated adenomas with BRAF mutations: a prospective study of patients undergoing colonoscopy. *Gastroenterology.* 2006;131(5):1400-1407.
15. Jass JR. Hyperplastic polyps of the colorectum–innocent or guilty? *Dis Colon Rectum.* 2001;44(2):163-166.

11

MY PATIENT WAS FOUND TO HAVE ABOUT 50 HYPERPLASTIC POLYPS RANGING FROM 5 TO 15 MM. WHAT CONDITION DO I NEED TO THINK ABOUT AND HOW SHOULD I MANAGE THIS PATIENT?

Christopher S. Huang, MD
Francis A. Farraye, MD, MSc
Michael J. O'Brien, MD, MPH

Your patient likely has a rare condition known as hyperplastic polyposis syndrome, or HPS. The World Health Organization has established the following criteria for the diagnosis of HPS[1]: (1) at least 5 hyperplastic polyps located proximal to the sigmoid colon, of which 2 are larger than 10 mm in diameter; or (2) any number of hyperplastic polyps located proximal to the sigmoid colon in an individual who has a first-degree relative with HPS; or (3) more than 30 hyperplastic polyps of any size, distributed throughout the colon. It should be noted that these criteria are somewhat arbitrary, and it is likely that when the underlying molecular and genetic mechanisms are better understood, improved diagnostic criteria can be established. In a recent review, Jass proposed that at least 2 distinct HPSs exist.[2] Type 1 is associated with multiple, proximally located hyperplastic polyps that are large and frequently BRAF-mutated, with endpoint carcinomas that have high levels of microsatellite instability (MSI) and/or CpG island methylation. Type 2 HPS is associated with numerous, small, distally located hyperplastic polyps that are frequently KRAS-mutated; Type 2 HPS has a significantly weaker association with colon cancer.

HPS is important because it is considered a premalignant condition. Although the true risk of colon cancer in HPS is not known, there are several case series reporting an incidence exceeding 50%.[3] Patients with HPS (Type 1) frequently harbor multiple and large hyperplastic polyps, in addition to other serrated polyps, such as sessile serrated adenomas (SSA, an atypical hyperplastic polyp variant), dysplastic serrated polyps (serrated adenomas and admixed polyps), and adenomas that have the phenotype of conventional adenomatous polyps. The endpoint carcinomas in the setting of HPS are heterogeneous, depending on their underlying pathogenesis. Some cancers in HPS are microsatellite stable (MSS), similar to those that arise via the traditional adenoma-carcinoma sequence characterized by a gatekeeper APC mutation and subsequent chromosomal deletions (loss of heterozygosity).[4] However, a substantial proportion of cancers in HPS (approximately 70%)[5] likely arise by way of an alternative pathway to malignancy now known as the "serrated pathway." In the serrated pathway, hyperplastic polyps, notably the SSA variant, represent the precursor lesions (as opposed to conventional adenomas), which have the potential to progress to dysplastic serrated polyps (serrated adenomas), and ultimately to cancer. These cancers have high levels of CpG island methylation, and are frequently (but not invariably) microsatellite instability (MSI). They are located predominantly in the proximal colon, and frequently show BRAF mutation, reflecting their origin in serrated polyps. The serrated pathway also has a second arm, the so-called "mild mutator" pathway, that is associated with low levels of CpG island methylation and a loss of heterozygosity of suppressor genes, culminating in tumors that show features of MSS and MSI-Low cancers.

Management of patients with HPS can be challenging, particularly if the polyp burden is significant. If possible, the gastroenterologist should quantify the number of polyps, and submit all polyps for histologic examination. It may be impossible and impractical to remove every polyp in a single session, especially diminutive hyperplastic polyps in the distal colon and rectum. However, special attention should be paid to patients who have polyps with certain "high-risk" features, such as large size (>10 mm) and location in the proximal colon. In addition, polyps that are subtle, sessile or flat, "fold-like" in appearance, and covered by a layer of mucusSSAs warrant special attention and should be completely resected, as these may represent sessile serrated adenomas. Clearly, all polyps that have the endoscopic appearance of conventional adenomas should also be removed in their entirety. Data regarding surveillance are severely lacking, but investigators have empirically recommended a 1- to 3- year surveillance interval, depending on the number, size, and histology of polyps, as well as the ability to remove or ablate both the hyperplastic and adenomatous polyps.[6] Colectomy may be justified in patients with an extremely high polyp burden, concomitant dysplastic serrated polyps, or multiple advanced adenomas. Finally, screening of first-degree relatives should be recommended, independent of the presence or absence of cancer in the patient with HPS. The appropriate age for commencement of screening relatives, and the screening interval, have not been established, although starting at age 40 years, or 10 years earlier than the earliest age at diagnosis in the family, has been recommended.[7]

References

1. Burt R, Jass J. Hyperplastic polyposis. In: Hamilton SR, Aaltonen LA, eds. *WHO International Classification of Tumors* (3rd ed). Lyon, France: IARC Press; 2000:135-136.
2. Jass JR. Gastrointestinal polyposes: clinical, pathological and molecular features. *Gastroenterol Clin North Am.* 2007;36(4):927-946.
3. Rubio CA, Stemme S, Jaramillo E, Lindblom A. Hyperplastic polyposis coli syndrome and colorectal carcinoma. *Endoscopy.* 2006;38(3):266-270.
4. Hawkins NJ, Gorman P, Tomlinson IP, Bullpitt P, Ward RL. Colorectal carcinomas arising in the hyperplastic polyposis syndrome progress through the chromosomal instability pathway. *Am J Pathol.* 2000;157(2):385-392.
5. Jass JR, Iino H, Ruszkiewicz A, et al. Neoplastic progression occurs through mutator pathways in hyperplastic polyposis of the colorectum. *Gut.* 2000;47(1):43-49.
6. Ferrández A, Samowitz W, DiSario JA, Burt RW. Phenotypic characteristics and risk of cancer development in hyperplastic polyposis: case series and literature review. *Am J Gastroenterol.* 2004;99(10):2012-2018.
7. Chow E, Lipton L, Lynch E, et al. Hyperplastic polyposis syndrome: phenotypic presentations and the role of MBD4 and MYH. *Gastroenterology.* 2006;131(1):30-39.

SECTION II

CONSTIPATION

What Should I Suspect When I See Melanosis Coli and What Is Its Clinical Relevance?

Erica Roberson, MD
Arnold Wald, MD

Melanosis coli is a dark brown-black discoloration of the colonic mucosa most often seen with exposure to anthraquinone laxatives (Figure 12-1). It is usually more prominent in the proximal colon and cecum, although it can affect the entire large bowel. Up to 70% of patients who use anthraquinone laxatives chronically will develop melanosis coli within 4 to 12 months of starting the drug. It is therefore often seen in women aged 20 to 70 (the population most often affected with constipation), but its development does not depend on age or duration of constipation. Anthraquinone laxatives encompass cascara sagrada, senna, aloe, rhubarb, and frangula. Senna is the only anthraquinone approved by the Food and Drug Administration. The others are plant substances that may be found in products sold in homeopathic and nutritional stores. Melanosis coli has also been described uncommonly with other conditions including inflammatory bowel disease and diverticulosis and with medications including bisacodyl, topical anthralin, and bamboo leaf oil.

Melanosis coli is more accurately called pseudomelanosis coli since it is actually associated with lipofuscin, which is not melanin or a melanin-like substance. Lipofuscin is a marker for colonic epithelial cell apoptosis. Anthraquinone-containing laxatives are converted to active compounds by colonic bacteria, which induce apoptosis of colon epithelial cells. Cell remnants are then ingested by macrophages that migrate to the lamina propria where lysosymes convert remnants of cells into residual bodies containing the black pigment lipofuscin.[1]

In a patient who complains of chronic diarrhea, melanosis coli observed on colonoscopy is virtually diagnostic for surreptitious anthraquinone laxative use (factitious diarrhea). This could be deliberate or accidental through the use of over-the-counter supplements that contain anthraquinones. Melanosis coli is benign and reversible; stopping the offend-

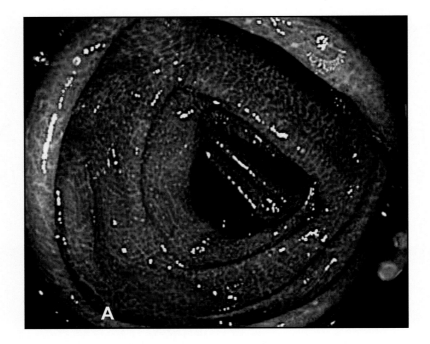

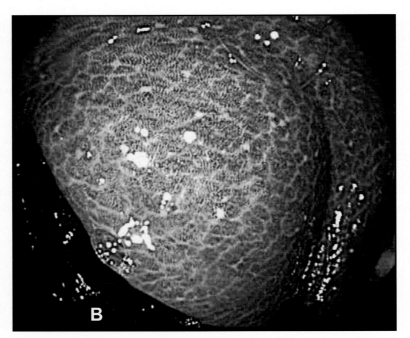

Figure 12-1. Melanosis coli is demonstrated by diffuse black pigment in the colonic mucosa (A). A close-up of anthraquinone-induced melanosis coli (B).

ing agent results in resolution within 4 to 12 months. There is no relationship between melanosis coli and colon cancer. In fact, neoplasms often can be identified more easily as they are nonpigmented and highlighted against the diffusely pigmented background.[2] There is no evidence that melanosis coli causes changes in colonic motility or secretion or that it has any physiologic importance.[3]

References

1. Wald A. Constipation and constipation syndromes. In: Weinstein WM, Hawkey CJ, Bosch J, eds. *Clinical Gastroenterology and Hepatology: Diseases of the Gut and Liver.* Philadelphia, PA: Elselvier, Inc; 2005:443-452.
2. Nascimbeni R, Donato F, Ghirardi M, Mariani P, Villanacci V, Salerni B. Constipation, anthranoid laxatives, melanosis coli, and colon cancer: a risk assessment using aberrant crypt foci. *Cancer Epidemiol Biomarkers Prev.* 2002;11(8):753-757.
3. Villanacci V, Bassotti G, Cathomas G, et al. Is pseudomelanosis coli a marker of colonic neuropathy in severely constipated patients? *Histopathology.* 2006;49(2):132-137.

What Should Be the Sequence of Investigations for a Patient Who Is Being Considered for Colectomy Due to Chronic Constipation?

Erica Roberson, MD
Arnold Wald, MD

Colectomy is an important treatment option for severe, intractable constipation in a small percentage of patients with exclusive colon dysmotility not responsive to medical treatment. As such, patients should be carefully selected in order to increase the chances of a successful outcome from this surgery. Patients who will benefit most are those with lifestyle-altering constipation from colonic inertia, without generalized dysmotility of the remaining gastrointestinal tract and without anorectal dysfunction.

Symptoms of constipation alone do not distinguish patients with colonic inertia, which is defined as (1) severe, unremitting constipation, (2) absence of a defecation disorder, (3) delayed passage of radiopaque markers in the proximal colon without evidence of retropulsion of markers in the left colon, and (4) no increase in colon motor activity in response to food, cholinergic agents, or stimulant laxatives.

Our understanding of the pathophysiology underlying colonic inertia has only recently been deciphered. Baseline colonic motility appears to be normal, however no increase in colonic activity is seen in response to known stimuli such as eating, cholinergic agents, and stimulant laxatives. Histologic studies suggest enteric neuronal loss, specifically, a decrease in enteric neurons, interstitial cells of Cajal (ICC), and enteric glial cells (EGC). ICC are the intestinal "pacemakers," and EGC are support cells that form the myelin sheath around axons and maintain appropriate concentrations of neurotransmitters.[1]

A 2-week bowel diary should initially be obtained to evaluate bowel patterns and habits together with a colonic transit study to provide objective evidence for normal or slow transit through the colon. Methods of performing this test vary among centers, but the general concept is this: radiopaque markers are swallowed and 1 or 2 x-rays are performed over the following 5 to 7 days. In patients with normal transit, the number of markers that remain in the colon is within the range established in normal control subjects; patients with slow transit have retention of more markers, and these may vary with regard to their distribution in the colon. Slow transit can be produced by either colonic inertia or a defecation disorder; therefore, patients with slow transit should undergo further evaluation to distinguish between these two entities.

One simple and inexpensive test of defecation that can be done in the office is the balloon expulsion test. In the presence of a significant defecation disorder, the patient likely will not be able to expel a 50-mL water-filled balloon within 60 seconds. If the patient can expel the balloon within 60 seconds, it is likely that a defecation disorder is not present (negative predictive value 97%).

If the balloon expulsion test is abnormal, the patient should be referred for anorectal manometry. This test will provide information on rectal sensation and compliance, relaxation of the internal anal sphincter, and manometric patterns of expulsion. Normally, a patient will have increased intrarectal pressures and decreased anal sphincter pressure when asked to expel the manometer. However, if a defecation disorder is present, anal sphincter pressure will either increase or not decrease during attempted expulsion of the manometer. This test should be normal if colectomy is being considered for colonic inertia.[2]

Finally, it is important to perform (1) esophageal manometry, (2) gastric emptying, and (3) small bowel motility studies to attempt to exclude a generalized gastrointestinal motility disorder, because the presence of generalized gastrointestinal dysmotility is associated with poor outcome after subtotal colectomy.

In summary, patients with constipation are candidates for colectomy if they have proven refractory colonic inertia with normal anorectal function, do not have abdominal pain as a major complaint, and do not have evidence of generalized GI tract dysmotility. The surgery of choice is a subtotal colectomy with ileorectal anastomosis. If both a defecation disorder and colonic inertia are present and the defecation disorder is not responsive to biofeedback therapy, a colectomy with ileostomy or sigmoid colostomy may be considered.

References

1. Bassotti G, Villanacci V. Slow transit constipation: a functional disorder becomes an enteric neuropathy. *World J Gastroenterol.* 2006;12(29):4609-4613.
2. Wald A. Chronic constipation: advances in management. *Neurogastroenterol Motil.* 2007;19(1):4-10.

WHAT DO I TELL MY PRIMARY CARE COLLEAGUES ABOUT CHRONIC CONSTIPATION AND THE RISK OF COLORECTAL CANCER?

Erica Roberson, MD
Arnold Wald, MD

Chronic constipation has been shown to be a small, albeit significant, risk for colon cancer.[1,2] Although poorly understood, this may have to do with increased concentration and colon residence of presumed carcinogens. Several studies have evaluated the possible link between colon cancer and chronic constipation and laxative use with conflicting conclusions. A recent meta-analysis of 14 case-control studies concluded that constipation and the use of cathartics is associated with an increased risk of developing colon cancer with pooled odds ratios of 1.48 (1.32 to 1.66) and 1.46 (1.33 to 1.61), respectively.[3] These odds ratios are significantly less than various dietary habits, such as high consumption of fats, meats, alcohol, and low residue diets, all of which are associated with odds ratios of 2 to 4 for the development of colon cancer. So it is entirely possible that the increased risk of colon cancer in this meta-analysis reflects the confounding influence of dietary habits. In one case-control study performed on middle-aged adults, both cathartics and chronic constipation were associated with an increased risk of colon cancer; however, after these variables were adjusted for each other, the risk only remained for constipation. This finding was confirmed in a larger, population-based case-control investigation.

It is important to realize, however, that studies have shown that the overall detection of colorectal cancer or adenomas is similar in patients with constipation compared to nonconstipated patients undergoing screening colonoscopy. In fact, the American College of Gastroenterology's position is that chronic constipation is not an indication for colonoscopy unless alarm symptoms exist (hematochezia, weight loss, family history, inflammatory bowel disease, anemia, positive fecal occult blood tests).[4] If a patient older than 50 years presents for evaluation of constipation, this is certainly an opportune time to encourage age-appropriate screening for colorectal cancer.[5]

The risk of cancer associated with laxatives has been a controversial topic. Very high doses of diphenylmethane laxatives (10 to 1000 times the doses used in humans) were shown to be carcinogenic in animal models (although not associated with colon cancer per se); this resulted in the removal of phenolphthalein from the US over-the-counter (OTC) market by the Food and Drug Administration. Many anthraquinones were also voluntarily removed from the OTC market because of fears of a possible link between these agents and colon cancer. However, large case-control studies suggest that these medications do not increase the risk of colon cancer in humans. Further studies have confirmed that anthraquinone laxatives and bisacodyl are safe at prescribed doses. Finally, melanosis coli, a common finding in patients taking certain laxatives, has not been associated with an increased risk of colon cancer.[6]

References

1. Jacobs EJ, White E. Constipation, laxative use, and colon cancer among middle-aged adults. Epidemiology. 1998;9(4):385-391.
2. Roberts MC, Millikan RC, Galanko JA, et al. Constipation, laxative use, and colon cancer in a North Carolina population. *Am J Gastroenterol.* 2003;98(4):857-864.
3. Sonnenberg A, Muller AD. Constipation and cathartics as risk factors for colorectal cancer: a meta-analysis. *Pharmacology.* 1993;47(suppl 1):224-233.
4. American College of Gastroenterology Chronic Constipation Task Force. An evidence-based approach to the management of chronic constipation in North America. *Am J Gastroenterol.* 2005;100(suppl 1):S1-S4.
5. Pepin C, Ladabaum U. The yield of lower endoscopy in patients with constipation: survey of a university hospital, a public county hospital, and a Veterans Administration medical center. *Gastrointest Endosc.* 2002;56(3):325-332.
6. Muller-Lissner SA, Kamm MA, Scarpignato C, Wald A. Myths and misconceptions about chronic constipation. *Am J Gastroenterol.* 2005;100(1):232-242.

WHAT DIAGNOSTIC TESTS ARE RECOMMENDED FOR THE EVALUATION OF CHRONIC CONSTIPATION AND WHAT IS THEIR YIELD?

Erica Roberson, MD
Arnold Wald, MD

Constipation is a very common disorder with prevalence rates in the United States as high as 28%. Despite the frequency of constipation in the general population, it is usually mild, intermittent, and often self-medicated with readily available over-the-counter medications. When patients with constipation present to a physician, an extensive workup is neither obligatory, nor justified, without alarm symptoms (anemia, weight loss, blood in stools, abdominal mass, nausea, vomiting, anorexia, an acute change in bowel movement) or when clinical judgment deems it necessary. The initial approach generally entails empirically treating constipation with little or no workup.[1]

The symptoms of chronic constipation do not reliably distinguish among the causes of constipation. Therefore, if constipation does not respond to medical treatment, further workup should entail evaluation of colonic and anorectal function with consideration of referral to a gastroenterology specialist.

Initial evaluation of refractory constipation begins with a colonic transit study (Figure 15-1). This study involves ingestion of radio-opaque markers with subsequent x-rays at set time points and quantification of markers remaining in the colon. Normal colonic transit is present in at least 60% of patients referred to gastroenterologists, whereas slow colonic transit time may arise from either colonic dysmotility or a defecation disorder. This is an important diagnostic consideration as the latter often responds to biofeedback therapy.

A balloon expulsion test is a useful next step. It measures the patient's ability to expel a 50-mL water-filled balloon and is done in the privacy of a restroom. A positive test should be followed by anorectal manometry to determine if there is a manometric abnormality to

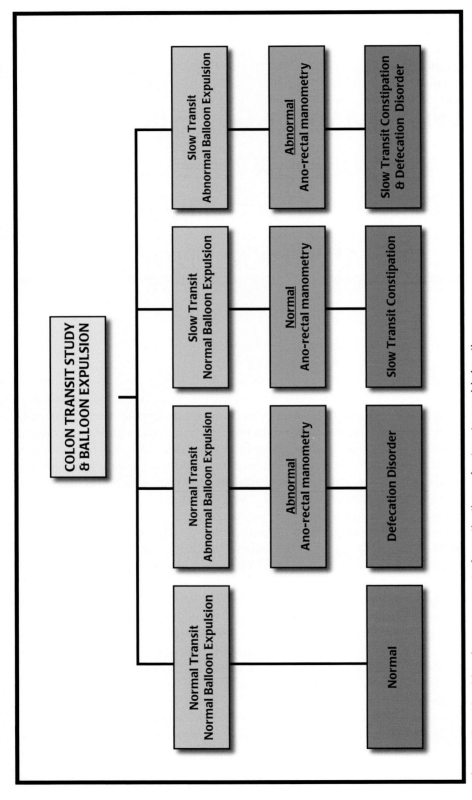

Figure 15-1. Algorithm for assessment of constipation refractory to empiric laxatives.

explain why the balloon cannot be expelled. If both tests are positive, the patient should undergo biofeedback treatment for a defecation disorder.[2]

If there is no evidence of a defecation disorder and the patient exhibits slow colonic transit, a diagnosis of colonic inertia is made. Most patients with this disorder may be managed successfully with laxatives and enterokinetic agents, often in combination. In a small number of patients, subtotal colectomy and ileorectal anastomosis may be considered if the patient is refractory to available agents and is disabled by the constipation.

References

1. American College of Gastroenterology Chronic Constipation Task Force. An evidence-based approach to the management of chronic constipation in North America. *Am J Gastroenterol.* 2005;100(suppl 1):S1-S4.
2. Rao SS, Ozturk R, Laine L. Clinical utility of diagnostic tests for constipation in adults: a systematic review. *Am J Gastroenterol.* 2005;100(7):1605-1615.

How Efficacious Are the Therapies for Chronic Constipation? I Have Heard About Several New Drugs for Constipation—Have They Been Shown to Be Cost Effective?

Erica Roberson, MD
Arnold Wald, MD

The first choice of many patients for constipation is often fiber supplements (bulking agents), which are readily available in some foods or as over-the-counter preparations. Although a deficiency of dietary fiber uncommonly causes constipation, some individuals do respond to an increase in fiber to 20 to 30 g daily. Fiber has been shown to increase stool weight and decrease transit time through the gastrointestinal tract. Soluble fibers such as psyllium may be better tolerated than insoluble fibers, but this is highly variable. Patients should be told that immediate results are not to be expected, and the dose should be increased slowly over 1 to 2 weeks. Fiber should be used cautiously in patients with irritable bowel syndrome (IBS) as these patients may experience increased symptoms, including bloating and cramping. Fiber should be avoided in patients with megacolon, megarectum, colonic inertia, and defecation disorders.

If fiber supplements are ineffective, osmotic laxatives may be tried. These drugs work by retaining fluid in the gut lumen by osmotic forces. Magnesium-containing agents are usually the first choice because they are inexpensive and readily available without a prescription. However, one should be cautious about using them in patients with renal insufficiency. Nonabsorbable sugars (lactulose, sorbitol) are degraded by colonic bacteria to low molecular weight acids that function to osmotically retain fluid in the lumen. These may produce increased gas and bloating as a byproduct. These side effects are less prominent with polyethylene glycol (PEG), which is not degraded

---

Table 16-1
30-Day Cost of Common Laxatives[1]

Laxative	Cost
Senna	$2.70
Bisacodyl	$7.47
Milk of magnesium	$11.40
Psyllium	$11.40 - 34.20
Sorbitol	$21.00
Polyethylene glycol	$34.16
Lactulose	$40.02
Tegaserod	Restricted access
Lubiprostone	$207.98

---

by intracolonic bacteria. Osmotic laxatives should be used daily and titrated to best effect. They may, however, be both ineffective and counterproductive in patients with colonic inertia and megacolon.

Stimulant laxatives such as senna (anthraquinones) and bisacodyl (diphenylmethanes) are time-honored agents that work by increasing luminal fluid accumulation and stimulating colonic motor activity. They have been unfairly criticized as causing cancer, producing laxative addiction and dependency, and harming the colon if used for long periods of time. These allegations have not been substantiated. Stimulant laxatives are often cost effective and produce satisfactory results in many patients. They can be given alone or in addition to bulking or osmotic agents.[2]

The Food and Drug Administration (FDA) has approved two newer agents for chronic constipation in the past few years. The first is tegaserod, a partial serotonin 5-HT$_4$ agonist, which acts to facilitate gastrointestinal motility. More recently released was lubiprostone, which works by stimulating specific intestinal chloride channels (ClC-2) and therefore increasing intestinal fluid secretion. Both drugs have been shown to be effective compared to placebo, but neither should be a first-line agent as they are quite expensive. In March 2007, the makers of tegaserod, in conjunction with the FDA, voluntarily suspended sales and marketing of the agent after a review of clinical trial data indicated that tegaserod may be associated with an increased risk of cardiovascular adverse events, such as angina pectoris, myocardial infarction, and cerebrovascular accidents. Tegaserod has been made available through a treatment investigational new drug program administered by the manufacturer and the FDA for women younger than age 55 who meet specific criteria with regard to their cardiovascular risk factors and symptoms of IBS-C and chronic idiopathic constipation.[3]

No trial or meta-analysis has yet demonstrated that one laxative is more effective than another or that lubiprostone or tegaserod are better than less expensive agents (Table 16-1). A reasonable approach is to start with a fiber supplement and add or switch to an osmotic and/or stimulant laxative if the response is unsatisfactory. If this regimen does not relieve constipation, use of tegaserod or lubiprostone with a possible referral to a gastroenterologist for further evaluation should be considered.

References

1. www.drugstore.com. Accessed July 31, 2008.
2. Brandt LJ, Prather CM, Quigley EM, Schiller LR, Schoenfeld P, Talley NJ. Systematic review on the management of chronic constipation in North America. *Am J Gastroenterol.* 2005;100 (suppl 1):S5-S21.
3. Wald A. Chronic constipation: advances in management. *Neurogastroenterol Motil.* 2007;19(1):4-10.

WHEN SHOULD A PATIENT COMPLAINING OF CHRONIC CONSTIPATION BE SENT FOR ANORECTAL MANOMETRY?

Erica Roberson, MD
Arnold Wald, MD

Patients who have failed conservative laxative therapy for constipation should undergo further evaluation, as symptoms alone do not determine underlying pathophysiology. Anorectal manometry is a helpful test to obtain as it provides insight on anorectal contributions to constipation (Figure 17-1). Specifically, manometry provides information about rectal motor and sensation functions to determine if a functional defecation disorder, such as dyssynergic defecation, or Hirschsprung disease is the cause of chronic constipation in patients who have failed conservative therapy.[1]

Disordered defecation can result from inappropriate contraction of the external anal sphincter and puborectalis muscle (Type I dyssynergia), absence of relaxation of those muscles (Type II), or impaired expulsion during attempted defecation (see Figure 17-1).[2] These result in insufficient forces to empty the rectum. However, at least 20% to 30% of patients with a dyssynergic pattern on anorectal manometry will have normal defecation, which is likely secondary to the artificial setting under which anorectal testing is performed in the laboratory. Therefore, a positive anorectal manometry test requires a confirmatory study, such as balloon expulsion, which measures the time to expel a rectal balloon filled with 50 mL of water (normal <60 sec). If both anorectal manometry and balloon expulsion are normal, a defecation disorder is very unlikely. If only one of these tests is positive, a third study, such as defecography, should be obtained. The importance of such testing is to diagnose a defecation disorder, which is often amenable to biofeedback therapy.[3]

As most patients do not have Hirschsprung as the etiology of their constipation, manometry is a relatively noninvasive way to exclude the diagnosis by demonstrating internal anal sphincter (IAS) relaxation in response to rectal distension (Figure 17-2). If

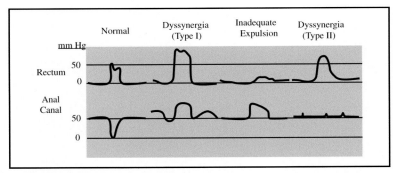

Figure 17-1. Manometry of the rectum and anal canal demonstrating 3 patterns of disordered defecation compared to normal. Type I is adequate abdominal pressures with inappropriate anal contraction; inadequate expulsion is weak or nonexistent propulsion with inappropriate contraction or no relaxation of the anal sphincter; and Type II is adequate propulsive with minimal or no anal relaxation.

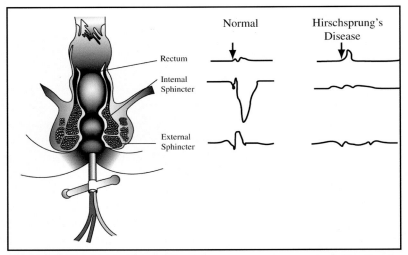

Figure 17-2. Anorectal manometry in a patient demonstrating inadequate relaxation of the internal sphincter during attempted defecation.

manometry shows absence of IAS relaxation, deep rectal biopsies must be obtained for histological evidence to confirm a diagnosis of Hirschsprung disease as technical issues are often the reason for failure to demonstrate relaxation of the IAS.

References

1. Sun WM, Rao SS. Manometric assessment of anorectal function. *Gastroenterol Clin North Am.* 2001;30(1):15-32.
2. Rao SS, Mudipalli RS, Stessman M, Zimmerman B. Investigation of the utility of colorectal function tests and rome II criteria in dyssynergic defecation (anismus). *Neurogastroenterol Motil.* 2004;16(5):589-596.
3. Bharucha AE, Wald A, Enck P, Rao S. Functional anorectal disorders. *Gastroenterology.* 2006;130(5):1510-1518.

A PATIENT ASKS ABOUT BIOFEEDBACK THERAPY FOR HER CONSTIPATION SYMPTOMS AND WANTS TO KNOW WHAT IS INVOLVED. WHAT DO I TELL HER?

Erica Roberson, MD
Arnold Wald, MD

Biofeedback is an effective therapy specifically for chronic constipation secondary to dyssynergic defecation. Normal defecation involves a coordinated cascade of events: intra-abdominal pressures increase while anal canal pressures decrease and pelvic floor muscles relax in order to widen the anorectal angle. In some patients, the anal sphincters do not relax or actually contract, resulting in an increase in anal canal pressure, the puborectalis muscle does not relax or actually contracts to narrow the anorectal angle, and/or inadequate intra-abdominal pressures are generated. Dyssynergic defecation is a relatively new concept and has been given a variety of names including pelvic floor dysfunction, pelvic floor dyssynergia, and outlet obstruction.

Biofeedback therapy is an effective and durable treatment in 70% to 80% of patients with documented dyssynergic defecation and is more effective than laxative use. Several studies have shown that, compared to standard medical therapy with laxatives or to sham biofeedback, patients with dyssynergic defecation treated with biofeedback therapy have subjective improvement in their constipation symptoms as well as objective improvement in stool frequency, laxative use, straining, and bloating.[1] Candidates for this therapy should undergo balloon expulsion studies and anorectal manometry to establish the diagnosis before being offered this option. There is no evidence that biofeedback therapy helps patients with normal-transit constipation, irritable bowel syndrome with constipation, colonic inertia, or secondary constipation.[2]

Biofeedback works to improve coordination of the pelvic floor. Perception and response to rectal distension are developed, as well as the muscular relaxation of the pelvic floor. These functions are controlled partially at a cortical level, which allows them to be altered with conscious efforts. Biofeedback works by providing visual feedback in the form of pressure recordings or electromyograph tracings to patients. Training sessions last approximately 30 to 45 minutes and are provided weekly or several times per week until coordination is established, or until treatment is deemed unsuccessful. Biofeedback is performed similarly to anorectal manometry with a pressure-sensitive balloon placed into the rectum and connected to various transducers capable of displaying pressure tracings on a screen or tracing paper. First, patients are taught to strain more effectively and coordinate expulsion efforts with breathing. Then, the patient is taught to relax the pelvic floor muscles and sphincter while straining. Finally, patients practice defecating and are given positive feedback. With visual feedback and practice, the patient is able to learn the physical skills of perceiving rectal distension and relaxing pelvic floor muscles while straining to defecate. As biofeedback often results in good outcomes, including improved quality of life, and it entails no risks, this behavioral therapy should be the first line of therapy in patients found to have dyssynergic defecation.

References

1. Chiarioni G, Whitehead WE, Pezza V, Morelli A, Bassotti G. Biofeedback is superior to laxatives for normal transit constipation due to pelvic floor dyssynergia. *Gastroenterology.* 2006;130(3):657-664.
2. Chiarioni G, Salandini L, Whitehead WE. Biofeedback benefits only patients with outlet dysfunction, not patients with isolated slow transit constipation. *Gastroenterology.* 2005;129(1):86-97.

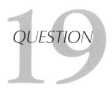

WHAT ARE THE EMERGING THERAPEUTIC AGENTS FOR CONSTIPATION AND HOW DO THEY MODULATE COLONIC MOTILITY?

Brooks D. Cash, MD, FACP, FACG

The enteric nervous system (ENS) contains as many neurons as the spinal cord, which are spatially distributed along the digestive tract in close proximity to effector organs (smooth muscle, glandular epithelium), allowing for rapid, automatic feedback control. Interneurons and motor neurons are interconnected by chemical synapses to comprise functional neural networks that receive synaptic input from sensory neurons that detect changes in the thermal, chemical, or mechanical local environment.[1] Understanding the functional basis of the ENS, especially with respect to motility and secretion, is crucial for achieving a better understanding of how to manage patients with chronic constipation (Figure 19-1).

Motor neurons in the ENS fall into 2 broad categories: excitatory or inhibitory. Excitatory motor neurons promote contraction of the gastrointestinal tract smooth muscle and secretion from mucosal glands. The primary excitatory neurotransmitters involved in muscle contraction include acetylcholine and substance P. Inhibitory motor neurons release neurotransmitters that suppress contractile activity and secretion. These include vasoactive intestinal polypeptide, nitric oxide, and Adenosine-5'-triphosphate.[1,2] Gastrointestinal contractions may be classified on the basis of their duration. Short duration contractions are known as phasic contractions and sustained contractions are called tonic contractions. Tonic contractions play a primary role in organs with reservoir functions (stomach, colon) and sphincter function, whereas phasic contractions are critical for the mixing of gastrointestinal contents and propulsion of those contents in an aboral direction. Colonic motility patterns are also classified as segmental activity or propagated activity. Segmental activity consists of single bursts of arrhythmic, low amplitude contractions that create a pressure gradient that slowly pushes intestinal contents toward the

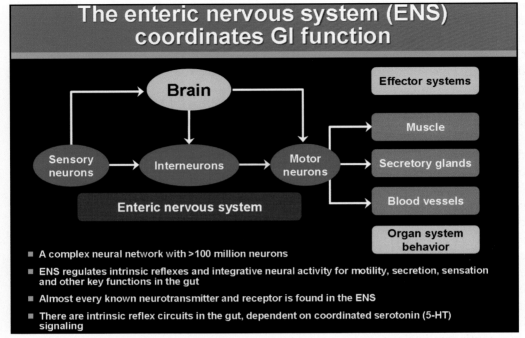

Figure 19-1. The integration of the enteric nervous system with the central nervous system and gastrointestinal tract. Adapted from Wood J. Neuropathophysiology of functional gastrointestinal disorders. *World J Gastroenterol.* 2007;13(9):1313-1332; and Gershon MD. Review article: serotonin receptors and transporters—roles in normal and abnormal gastrointestinal motility. *Aliment Pharmacol Ther.* 2004;20 Suppl 7:3-14.

rectum. Propagated activity occurs in the form of low amplitude propagated contractions (LAPC) or high amplitude propagated contractions (HAPC). LAPCs occur more than 100 times per day and are important for the transport of fluid within the colon.[3] HAPCs occur about 6 times per day and are the prototypical stripping waves that are involved in mass movements of fecal contents large distances within the colon. HAPCs are considered one of the driving forces behind defecation.[3] Dysfunctional gastrointestinal motility may arise through alterations of the control mechanisms at any level of the gut through to the central nervous system.

Secretion in the gastrointestinal tract is primarily mediated by secretomotor neurons that are located in the submucosal plexus of the ENS. They receive input from other ENS neurons (intrinsic nerves), as well as from sympathetic postganglionic nerves. Local paracrine messengers from non-neural cells such as enterochromaffin cells, mast cells, and other inflammatory cells can have a profound influence on the excitability of these secretomotor neurons. Excitatory input to secretomotor neurons is mediated by acetylcholine, vasoactive intestinal polypeptide, substance P, and serotonin. When stimulated, these neurons release acetylcholine and vasoactive intestinal polypeptide at both submucosal arterioles and intestinal glands. At the arterioles, acetylcholine promotes the release of nitric oxide to cause vasodilatation and at the intestinal crypt cells, Brunner's glands, and goblet cells, acetylcholine directly promotes the release of H_2O, NaCl, bicarbonate, and mucus into the intestinal lumen through specific channels as well as via passive diffusion. Inhibitory inputs include somatostatin-mediated messages from intrinsic ENS nerves and norepinephrine-mediated messages from postganglionic sympathetic nerves. Clinical examples of elevated secretomotor neuron activity include inflammatory bowel disease, in which inflammatory mediators excite the secretomotor neurons to release neurotransmitters and increase secretion, manifesting as diarrhea. Neuropathic conditions that diminish the functional or structural integrity of the ENS may be associated with diminished secretomotor neuron activity and may manifest as constipation.

Chloride and bicarbonate secretion provides 5 major physiologic functions in the digestive tract, including: 1) provision of an aqueous phase for digestion and absorption of meals, 2) hydration of mucus, 3) facilitation of the delivery of antibodies and cryptins (antimicrobial ligands) into the gut lumen, 4) helping to purge intestinal pathogens and noxious agents, and 5) adjusting luminal pH to optimize nutrient digestion and absorption.[4] Transporters that enable chloride secretion are located on the basolateral side of enterocytes. When chloride channels in the luminal or apical membrane open, active chloride secretion occurs, followed by passive diffusion of sodium and water. One of these channels is the cystic fibrosis transmembrane regulator (CFTR), which is highly regulated by second messengers. A second chloride transporter, the type 2 chloride channel (ClC-2), is also present in the luminal membrane. Therapeutic agents that can affect these channels have the potential to increase chloride and fluid secretion into the lumen and thus have therapeutic implications for patients with constipation.

Agents That Target GI Receptors in Constipation

Tegaserod, a partial 5-hydroxytryptamine (HT)$_4$ receptor agonist, is approved in the United States for the treatment of irritable bowel syndrome with constipation (IBS-C) in women, and chronic constipation in men and women younger than 65 years. Tegaserod accelerates transit by stimulating 5-HT$_4$ receptors in the ENS, thus increasing the release of proximal stimulatory and distal inhibitory neurotransmitters in the ENS, which in turn augments peristalsis. Tegaserod has been shown to improve the symptoms of constipation, bloating, and straining compared with placebo.[5] However, in March 2007, the manufacturer suspended marketing and sales of tegaserod because review of clinical trial data found that patients randomized to tegaserod had a higher risk of myocardial infarction, stroke, and unstable angina (heart/chest pain) compared with placebo. In April 2008, access to tegaserod was further restricted to emergency situations (defined as those that are immediately life-threatening or serious enough to warrant hospitalization).

Several mixed 5-HT$_4$ receptor agonists/5-HT$_3$ receptor antagonists are currently undergoing evaluation for the treatment of patients with symptomatic constipation. Camilleri and colleagues recently presented the combined results from 3 randomized double-blind trials showing that prucalopride was safe and effective at doses of 2 mg or 4 mg per day in patients with chronic idiopathic constipation.[6] For the 3 trials combined, 23.6% of patients in the 2-mg group and 24.7% of patients in the 4-mg group, compared with 11.3% in the placebo group, had an average of $\geq$3 spontaneous complete bowel movements per week over the 12-week treatment period ($P<.001$ for both dosage comparisons). Prucalopride has also demonstrated significant improvement over placebo in a phase 2, double-blind, placebo-controlled trial involving 180 patients with opioid-induced constipation.[7]

There are 5 different types of opiate receptors that have been found to modulate gut motor and sensory functions. Among these, mu receptor-avid agents have demonstrated the most promise as possible therapies for chronic constipation, specifically for patients with opioid-induced constipation. Alvimopan is a peripherally acting mu-opioid receptor antagonist that has been shown to selectively block the peripheral effects of morphine without appreciably decreasing its centrally-mediated analgesic effects and is currently FDA approved for the treatment of postoperative bowel dysfunction. It has been shown to accelerate colonic transit in healthy volunteers not taking opiates, and several phase 3 studies have demonstrated a clinically significant promotility effect of alvimopan in patients with postoperative ileus.[8,9] Another mu receptor antagonist, methylnaltrexone, is approved for the treatment of opioid-induced constipation. It is derived from the methylation of naltrexone, resulting in a molecule that does not readily cross the blood-brain barrier. A recently published phase 3 trial with methylnaltrexone in opioid-using patients with advanced illnesses showed that patients randomized to methylnaltrexone were 33% more likely to have defecation within 4 hours after at least 1 dose of methylnaltrexone.[10] An open-label extension study confirmed the persistence of the response and the absence of narcotic withdrawal symptoms.

Lubiprostone is a bicyclic fatty acid that selectively activates intestinal type-2 chloride channels on the apical intestinal membrane, thus increasing fluid secretion into the intestinal lumen. It is currently the only fully available prescription medication indicated for the treatment of chronic idiopathic constipation in the adult population. In clinical trials of lubiprostone, patients who received 24 mcg twice daily experienced significantly more spontaneous bowel movements than patients who received placebo (P<.002 at all weeks).[11,12] The most common side effect with this agent is nausea, which can be minimized when patients take lubiprostone with fluid and food.

Linaclotide is a potent guanylate cyclase-C agonist that acts peripherally to increase the production of cyclic guanosine monophosphate in human colon cells, leading to eventual activation of the CFTR to increase chloride, bicarbonate, and water secretion into the colon. Lembo recently presented the results of a phase 2b study involving 207 patients with chronic constipation who received 4 different doses of linaclotide over a 4-week period.[13] The intent-to-treat analysis showed that at doses greater than 75 mcg, patients experienced statistically significant improvements in complete spontaneous bowel movement frequency, as well as improvements in stool consistency, straining, bloating, and abdominal discomfort. The most common adverse event was diarrhea, which resulted in discontinuation in 3% of linaclotide-treated patients.

References

1. Wood J. Neuropathophysiology of functional gastrointestinal disorders. *World J Gastroenterol.* 2007;13(9):1313-1332.
2. Gershon MD. Review article: serotonin receptors and transporters—roles in normal and abnormal gastrointestinal motility. *Aliment Pharmacol Ther.* 2004;20 suppl 7:3-14.

3. Bassotti G, de Roberto G, Castellani D, Sediari L, Morelli A. Normal aspects of colorectal motility and abnormalities in slow transit constipation. *World J Gastroenterol.* 2005;11(18):2691-2696.
4. Harrell LE, Chang EB. Intestinal water and electrolyte transport. In: Feldman M, Friedman LS, Brandt LJ, eds. *Sleisenger & Fordtran's Gastrointestinal and Liver Disease.* 8th ed. Philadelphia, PA: Saunders; 2006:2127-2146.
5. Quigley EM, Wald A, Fidelholtz J, Boivin M, Pecher E, Earnest D. Safety and tolerability of tegaserod in patients with chronic constipation: pooled data from two phase III studies. *Clin Gastroenterol Hepatol.* 2006;49(5):605-613.
6. Camilleri M, Gryp RS, Kerstens R, et al. Efficacy of 12-week treatment with prucalopride (Resolor®) in patients with chronic constipation: combined results of three identical, randomized, double-blind, placebo-controlled phase 3 trials. *Gastroenterology.* 2008:134:suppl 1:A-548.
7. Moulin DE, Rykx A, Kerstens R, et al. Randomized, double-blind, placebo-controlled trial to evaluate efficacy and safety of prucalopride (Resolor®) in patients with opioid induced constipation. *Gastroenterology.* 2008:134:suppl 1 A-642.
8. Viscusi ER, Goldstein S, Witkowski T, et al. Alvimopan, a peripherally acting mu-opioid receptor antagonist, compared with placebo in postoperative ileus after major abdominal surgery: results of a randomized, double-blind, controlled study. *Surg Endosc.* 2006;20(1):64-70.
9. Delaney CP, Weese JL, Hyman NH, et al. Phase III trial of alvimopan, a novel, peripherally acting, mu opioid antagonist, for postoperative ileus after major abdominal surgery. *Dis Colon Rectum.* 2005;48(6):1114-1125.
10. Thomas J, Karver S, Cooney GA, et al. Methylnaltrexone for opioid-induced constipation in advanced illness. *N Engl J Med.* 2008;358(22):2332-2343.
11. Johanson JF, Gargano MA, Holland PC, et al. Initial and sustained effects of lubiprostone, a chloride channel-2 (CIC-2) activator for the treatment of constipation: data from a 4-week phase III study [abstract]. *Am J Gastroenterol.* 2005;100:S324–S325.
12. Johanson JF, Morton D, Geenen J, Ueno R. Multicenter, 4-week, double-blind, randomized, placebo-controlled trial of lubiprostone, a locally-acting type-2 chloride channel activator, in patients with chronic constipation. *Am J Gastroenterol.* 2008;103(1):170-177.
13. Lembo A. Linaclotide significantly improved bowel habits and relieved abdominal symptoms in adults with chronic constipation: data from a large four-week, randomized, double-blind, placebo-controlled study. *Gastroenterology.* 2008:134:suppl 1:P-100.

What Do I Tell My Colleagues Who Are Concerned About Neuropathic Changes From Laxative Use?

Richard Saad, MD

Laxatives are the most widely used medications in both the short- and long-term treatment of constipation. They are available by prescription as well as over-the-counter, and their primary therapeutic goal is to increase the frequency and ease of bowel movements. Laxatives work in a variety of ways within the gastrointestinal tract and are therefore categorized based on their mode of action. They are assigned to the stimulant, osmotic, bulk-forming, surfactant, or alternative/other categories.

Stimulant (irritant) laxatives alter electrolyte and fluid transport and/or bowel motility resulting in decreased fluid reabsorption and increased colonic/small bowel contractions. This includes diphenylmethanes (bisacodyl), anthraquinones (senna, danthorn, cascara, and aloe), castor oil, erythromycin, and misoprostol. They have been historically used in the treatment of acute constipation given their rapid onset of action, but are also used in the treatment of chronic constipation. Their efficacy at improving stool frequency and consistency remains largely anecdotal.[1] Common adverse effects include diarrhea, cramping, bloating, and nausea. Of all the classes of laxatives, stimulant laxatives have received the most attention and concern regarding the theoretical risk of enteric nervous system damage with their use.[2,3] Anthraquinone use is associated with a brown discoloration of the colon termed melanosis coli. This is due to staining of cell debris taken up by submucosal macrophages and is not known to have any functional significance. There are also conflicting reports of damage to the enteric nerves and smooth muscle in uncontrolled human observation studies and prospective animal studies.[2,3] Finally, there are reports of short-lived superficial mucosal changes with use of oral and rectal sodium phosphate and anthraquinones.[2] Although structural changes to surface epithelial cells can occur, there is no evidence that chronic stimulant laxative use leads to any structural or functional impairment of the enteric neuromuscular complex or function.

Osmotic agents are poorly absorbed substances that increase intraluminal water content, resulting in softer and bulkier stool. This class of laxatives includes milk of magnesia (magnesium hydroxide), polyethylene glycol (PEG) solutions, lactulose, and sorbitol. As a class, they are effective and well-tolerated medications in the treatment of constipation. PEG and lactulose are the best-studied osmotic laxatives with proven efficacy at increasing stool frequency, decreasing straining, and providing an overall benefit in constipation symptoms.[1] Side effects include electrolyte abnormalities, diarrhea, nausea, bloating, abdominal pain, and flatulence. Long-term safety studies are limited to a 6-month safety trial with PEG. There are no reports of any damage to the enteric nervous system with the use of these agents.

Bulking or hydrophilic laxative agents increase the weight and water absorbency of the stool. This class includes bran, psyllium, methylcellulose, ispaghula, celandine, and plantain derivatives. Their effectiveness in treating constipation is best demonstrated with psyllium, although results with the others are conflicting and high-quality studies are generally lacking.[1] Their side effect profile is minimal, including that of diarrhea, bloating, cramping, flatulence, and nausea. There are no reports of damage to the enteric nervous system with bulking agents.

Surfactant laxatives (stool softeners), such as docusate and poloxalkol, act as detergents to lubricate the stool in order to ease stool passage. There are limited studies assessing the effectiveness of these agents in the treatment of constipation with conflicting results.[1] Most authorities recommend against the use of stool softeners due to the paucity of evidence supporting their efficacy; however, their side effect profile is minimal and does not include the risk of damage to the enteric nervous system.

The alternative laxatives have a direct action on various receptors in the gastrointestinal tract promoting prosecretory and/or prokinetic effects. They remain among the best studied. Tegaserod is a selective 5-HT$_4$ (serotonin) receptor partial agonist. Serotonin is a neurotransmitter found in enteric nervous system modulating gut peristalsis, fluidity of the stool, and visceral sensation. Tegaserod improves the global symptoms associated with constipation through increases in spontaneous bowel movements, decreased straining, reduced bloating/distention, reduced abdominal pain/discomfort, and improved stool form.[1,4] Lubiprostone is a chloride-channel activator, acting selectively at the ClC-2 chloride channel on the apical surface of the intestinal mucosal epithelial cells. These receptors control the cell membrane transport of chloride ions. Activation of the ClC-2 receptor by lubiprostone increases the frequency of spontaneous bowel movements, improves stool consistency, and reduces straining.[5] Adverse effects include nausea, diarrhea, and headache. Long-term safety trials up to 12 months have been performed with both of these agents and there are no reports of enteric nervous system damage with either drug.

In summary, although laxatives are associated with variable side effects, there is no convincing evidence that their use either in the short- or long-term is associated with damage to the enteric neuromuscular system. Studies suggesting such damage with stimulant laxatives appear largely unfounded. Overall, laxatives have a favorable benefit-to-risk profile and have been time-tested as being safe and well tolerated.

References

1. Ramkumar D, Rao SS. Efficacy and safety of traditional medical therapies for chronic constipation: systematic review. *Am J Gastroenterol.* 2005;100(4):936-971.

2. Müller-Lissner SA, Kamm MA, Scarpignato C, Wald A. Myths and misconceptions about chronic constipation. *Am J Gastroenterol.* 2005;100(1):232-242.

3. Wald A. Is chronic use of stimulant laxatives harmful to the colon? *J Clin Gastroenterol.* 2003;36(5):386-389.

4. Kamm MA, Müller-Lissner S, Talley NJ, et al. Tegaserod for the treatment of chronic constipation: a randomized, double-blind, placebo-controlled multinational study. *Am J Gastroenterol.* 2005;100(2):362-372.

5. Johanson JF, Gargano MA, Patchen ML. Phase III efficacy and safety of RU-0211, a novel chloride channel activator, for the treatment of constipation [abstract]. *Gastroenterology.* 2003;124(suppl 1):A48.

SECTION III

DIARRHEA

WHAT COLONIC INFECTIONS ARE ASSOCIATED WITH AIDS?

Brian Mulhall, MD

Given the high-risk of infectious diarrhea in patients with human immunodeficiency virus, any patient with more than 1 week of diarrhea deserves appropriate workup.[1] Diarrhea is defined as more than 3 bowel movements and more than 200 g of stool output per day. Especially in patients with abdominal pain, large volume diarrhea, hematochezia, or fevers and chills, an infectious process has to be strongly considered. Stool samples should be sent for fecal leukocytes, stool culture, fecal ova and parasites (x 3), *Clostridium difficile* (especially in patients currently or recently on antibiotics, those with recent hospitalizations, or in those living in institutional settings), and acid-fast stains. Patients who appear systemically ill should be hospitalized and blood cultures should be performed.[1]

For AIDS patients with infectious diarrhea, a number of unusual culprit organisms need to be considered.[2] Organisms like *Mycobacterium avium*, *Cryptosporidium parvum*, and microspiridiae species are unique pathogens seen in the immunocompromised (Figure 21-1). However, more common organisms like *Clostridium difficile* and *Entamoeba histolytica* also deserve strong consideration. Bloody diarrhea should raise concerns for *Salmonella*, *Shigella*, and Enterohemorrhagic *E. Coli* (EHEC). Stool cultures and studies, to include assays for microsporidium and acid-fast organisms, can be essential in defining the etiology.

Of the various infectious diseases that can infect the colon in the setting of AIDS, one important consideration is cytomegalovirus (CMV). CMV is still an uncommon disorder, but is important to recognize because of the potential for morbidity and mortality if not diagnosed early. Historically, CMV infection of the gastrointestinal tract was thought to occur in up to about 5% of patients with AIDS, but the incidence of this infection has decreased as the rate of AIDS among patients with HIV has diminished through HAART (highly active antiretroviral therapy).[3] As the degree of viremia increases and the CD4 count decreases, the risk of CMV increases—as does the risk of other opportunistic infections of the intestinal tract. In addition to viremia and immunosuppression, the presence of CMV in the serum is the most important risk factor for gastrointestinal involvement. CMV colitis typically manifests with malaise, anorexia, weight loss, low-grade fevers,

Figure 21-1. An example of colonic cryptosporidiosis. Note the organisms within the crypts.

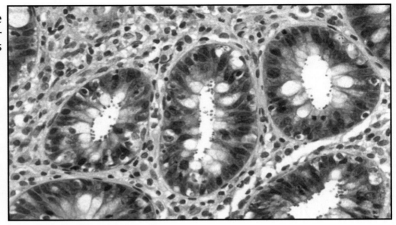

abdominal pain, and diarrhea.[4] Diarrhea can be episodic, but can also be quite severe and associated with life-threatening hemorrhage. Rarely, patients present with colonic perforation, which is the most devastating complication. Diagnosis is typically based on clinical suspicion, but can also be made though demonstration of CMV viremia or through CMV antigen assays. It should be noted, however, that AIDS patients can be viremic in the absence of colonic involvement, and CMV viremia may not be detectable in the setting of active CMV colitis. During endoscopic evaluation, the colon can range in appearance from normal to frank necrotizing colitis. Biopsies of the mucosa typically show inflammation, vascular endothelial infiltration, and tissue necrosis, but examination with hematoxylin and eosin staining should reveal large cells with eosinophilic and basophilic intracytoplasmic inclusion bodies called cytomegalic cells. Initiation of HAART therapy helps avoid the dreaded complications of hemorrhage and perforation. Before HAART therapy, infection of the colon with CMV carried a grim prognosis with nearly half of the patients dying within 4 months of diagnosis. Finally, it is important to recognize that patients infected with CMV colitis can often have concomitant CMV retinitis, so they should undergo ophthalmological assessment to address this possibility.

References

1. Mönkemüller KE, Wilcox CM. Diagnosis and treatment of colonic disease in AIDS. *Gastrointest Endosc Clin N Am.* 1998;8(4):889-911.
2. Johanson JF. Diagnosis and management of AIDS-related diarrhea. *Can J Gastroenterol.* 1996;10(7):461-468.
3. Thom K, Forrest G. Gastrointestinal infections in immunocompromised hosts. *Curr Opin Gastroenterol.* 2006;22(1):18-23.
4. Cheung TW, Teich SA. Cytomegalovirus infection in patients with HIV infection. *Mt Sinai J Med.* 1999; 66(2):113-124.

WE SEE MANY PATIENTS WITH BONE MARROW TRANSPLANTS. HOW DO WE RECOGNIZE AND TREAT GRAFT-VERSUS-HOST DISEASE IN THE COLON? HOW DO WE MAKE SURE WE ARE NOT MISSING CMV COLITIS?

Brian Mulhall, MD

Patients who have undergone allogeneic hematopoietic cell transplants (bone marrow transplants [BMT]) are more susceptible to gastrointestinal complications, like graft-versus-host disease (GVHD).[1] Diarrhea is relatively common after a BMT and can be related to medication side effects (ie, antibiotic-induced diarrhea), radiation side effects, infections, or GVHD. GVHD is most likely to affect the skin and the liver, but can have devastating effects when it impacts the gastrointestinal tract or the hematopoietic system. GVHD may occur with HLA-identical matches as well as with matched unrelated donors, but is more common in HLA-mismatches, in patients on higher doses of immunomodulators (cyclosporine, methotrexate, and tacrolimus), in patients with greater exposure to radiation, in older patients, and in gender-mismatched pairings. The more severe the GVHD, the more likely it will negatively impact survival after BMT.

Patients with gastrointestinal GVHD will characteristically present with abdominal pain and cramping, along with diarrhea.[1] They can also manifest with nausea/vomiting, weight loss, dysphagia, and early satiety. More rarely, they can be mildly symptomatic or even asymptomatic. The abdominal pain associated with GVHD is often quite intense, the diarrhea can be severe, and the fluid losses profound. Patients with GVHD may develop hemorrhagic diarrhea and require blood transfusions. Patients also need to be monitored for the development of colonic atony that can result from narcotics required for pain relief from the GVHD itself.

Early recognition of GVHD is critical to improving patient outcomes, but once acute GVHD occurs, it may not be reversible. The "gold standard" for diagnosis is a rectal biopsy. Studies that have looked at the diagnostic yield of endoscopy in the evaluation of acute intestinal GVHD found that the combination of upper endoscopy with sigmoid-oscopy compared to colonoscopy had equivalent yields.[1] Distal colon biopsies have the highest yield for making the diagnosis. In acute GVHD of the intestines, histology examination will show crypt cell necrosis or intra-cryptal apoptosis with or without cryptitis, and may show marked epithelial sloughing in more severe cases. In chronic GVHD of the intestines (which is much less common), fibrosis and crypt distortion is more likely to be seen. Because infection with cytomegalovirus (CMV) can present very similarly to colonic GVHD, it is always important to request that special staining is performed to rule out this possibility.[2] Specifically, the pathologist will be looking for viral inclusions in the case of CMV, but light microscopy alone may be inadequate. The addition of DNA in situ hybridization improves accuracy.

There have been several studies showing that noninvasive studies, like computed tomography scanning, can be useful in diagnosing acute GVHD of the intestines. Specifically, thickening of the distal esophagus, ileum, and ascending colon are predictive of high-grade GVHD. Nonetheless, confirmation by biopsy is warranted prior to treatment, given the other conditions that may mimic such nonspecific findings. Because early diagnosis and the initiation of corticosteroid therapy can improve outcomes, the distinction between infection and acute GVHD is especially important in BMT patients.

The standard regimen that is used most widely for prevention of GVHD is cyclosporine plus short-term methotrexate.[3] Corticosteroids can be added to this regimen but careful consideration of the adverse effects of these hormones should be considered. Tacrolimus, a more potent alternative to cyclosporine, is also commonly used. T-cell depletion (TCD) after transplantation has been shown to prevent acute GVHD, however, the survival benefit of TCD has not been as great as expected. Mycophenolate mofetil can be useful for the treatment of acute GVHD as part of combination therapy. Regimens currently under investigation in animal experiments include suppression of inflammatory cytokines and inhibition of T-cell activation, and hepatocyte growth factor gene therapy. Typical therapeutic regimens for intestinal GVHD include systemic antibacterial therapy in order to eradicate intestinal bacteria to prevent the intestinal translocation of lipopolysaccharide and avoid the subsequent increase of inflammatory cytokines. Because of the similarities between intestinal GVHD and ulcerative colitis, sulfasalazine, betamethasone enemas, and eicosapentaenoic acid have been used to treat intestinal GVHD in some patients.

References

1. Iqbal N, Salzman D, Lazenby AJ, Wilcox CM. Diagnosis of gastrointestinal graft-versus-host disease. *Am J Gastroenterol*. 2000;95(11):3034-3038.
2. Buckner FS, Pomeroy C. Cytomegalovirus disease of the gastrointestinal tract in patients without AIDS. *Clin Infect Dis*. 1993;17(4):644-656.
3. Takatsuka H, Iwasaki T, Okamoto T, Kakishita E. Intestinal graft-versus-host disease: mechanisms and management. *Drugs*. 2003;63(1):1-15.

MANY OF MY PATIENTS WANT TO GO WITH NATURAL THERAPIES. WHERE DO PROBIOTICS FIT IN THE MANAGEMENT OF IRRITABLE BOWEL SYNDROME?

Brooks D. Cash, MD, FACP, FACG

The literature regarding the use of probiotics in irritable bowel syndrome (IBS) has been fraught with methodological problems. Chief among these have been small sample size and a lack of consistency in the number, strain, and method of delivery of the probiotic agent(s).[1] Some studies have used a single purified strain of bacteria or yeast, whereas others have used a variety of probiotic "cocktails" with or without substrates designed to enhance the growth and viability of the organism. Various authors have confirmed an alteration in stool flora by performing quantitative stool cultures before and after therapy, whereas others have not. The World Health Organization and the Food and Agricultural Organization of the United Nations (WHO/FAO) define a probiotic as "live micro-organisms which, when administered in adequate amounts, confer a health benefit on the host."[2] The use of live microorganisms for purported health benefits, primarily as part of cultured milk products, dates back to at least the 7th century BC. The gastrointestinal tract, which is home to more than 500 different species of bacteria, has been the primary target of such remedies. Despite this long history, high-quality studies of the effects of probiotics on health and disease were not undertaken until the latter part of the past century.

The normal microbiota of the gut consists primarily of facultative anaerobes and obligate anaerobes, including *Bacteroides, Bifidobacterium, Clostridium, Enterobacter, Enterococcus, Escherichia, Eubacterium, Klebsiella, Lactobacillus, Peptococcus, Peptostreptococcus, Proteus,* and *Ruminococcus* species. These organisms perform numerous salutary functions, including metabolism of toxins, production of vitamins, and digestion of dietary products. Perhaps more importantly, they provide the first line of defense against colonization by pathogenic organisms. Given the complex relationship between our immune system and the endogenous microflora of our intestinal tracts, probiotics seem a "natural" choice as potentially therapeutic agents.

In 2004, Tsuchiya et al published data regarding the utility of the symbiotic mixture SCM-III in 68 consecutive adults with IBS.[3] SCM-III contains not only live bacteria (in this case *L. acidophilus, L. helviticus,* and *Bifidobacterium* species) but also specific substrates known as prebiotics that improve microbial growth and survival. Participants were given either 10 mL of SCM-III three times a day or a placebo composed of a heat-inactivated version of the same preparation. Patients were assessed for overall clinical status (primarily abdominal discomfort) and "bowel habits" (a subjective composite of stool frequency and consistency) at baseline, 3, 6, and 12 weeks. Abdominal pain and bloating were independently assessed at similar intervals. Eighty percent of the SCM-III patients versus only 15% of the control patients reported that the treatment was "effective" to "very effective." Nearly 40% of the placebo recipients felt SCM-III was "slightly effective," consistent with the placebo effect found in other IBS treatment trials. Although abdominal pain improved, no significant change in bloating in drug patients versus placebo patients was noted at 12 weeks. Several other investigators, however, have shown reductions in bloating in IBS patients using VSL#3 and *L. plantarum,* respectively.[4,5]

The most significant article on this topic was published by O'Mahony et al.[6] In this study, the investigators examined the effects of *L. salivarius* UCC4331 or *B. infantis* 35624 versus placebo in a randomized, double-blind trial of 77 IBS patients. What makes this study particularly intriguing is the assessment not only of the cardinal symptoms of IBS, but also of changes in the ratio of the interleukins IL-10 and IL-12 in peripheral blood mononuclear cells (PBMCs). IL-10 is the product of a number of immunomodulatory cells, including mast cells, B lymphocytes, Th1 and Th2 lymphocytes, and mononuclear phagocytic cells. It inhibits the production of interferons and interleukins, and TNF-α. *Bifidobacterium* has been associated with suppression of IFN-γ, TNF-α, and IL-12. Prior to probiotic administration, the authors examined the IL-10 and IL-12 levels of IBS patients and 20 asymptomatic controls. The levels of IL-12 were higher, and IL-10 lower, in the IBS patients, indicating a proinflammatory state. The subjects were then given *L. salivarius, B. infantis,* or placebo for 8 weeks and followed for a 4-week washout period. The subjects taking *B. infantis* enjoyed a significant decrease in all symptomatic parameters, including abdominal pain/discomfort, bloating/distention, and bowel movement difficulties. *L. salivarius* produced a result no different than that of placebo. Interestingly, the IL-10/IL-12 ratio normalized in those taking *B. infantis* but not in those taking *L. salivarius* or placebo despite participants achieving increased levels of *Lactobacillus* in their stools. This finding adds biologic plausibility that the changes in symptoms were indeed due to the *Bifidobacterium.*

In one of the longest trials to date, Niv et al performed a 6-month, double-blind, randomized, placebo-controlled trial of a single organism, *L. reuteri* ATCC 55730, in 54 IBS patients.[7] Patients all had significant symptoms at the onset of the study as measured by the Francis Severity Score (FSS) of greater than 75 (out of 100). Patients were followed for 6 months, and measured outcomes were changes in FSS and IBS-related quality of life. Thirty-nine patients completed the study, and no significant differences were noted between groups for changes in FSS or IBS quality of life. Although it is possible that a larger sample size might have revealed a subtle difference between the groups, this study provides compelling evidence for the lack of efficacy for this organism in IBS. Kim et al examined the utility of VSL#3 in a 4-week, double-blind, randomized, placebo-controlled trial in 48 IBS patients.[4] The primary symptomatic outcome measure was bloating severity. Flatulence, stool-related symptoms (ease of stool passage, stool frequency, and number of days with incomplete evacuation), abdominal pain, and satisfactory relief of bloating (defined as improved >50% of the weeks) were secondary symptomatic outcomes. No significant difference was seen in the primary outcome of bloating, though a statistically significant decrease in flatulence was noted.

Although the use of probiotics is still in its infancy, the literature regarding the use of probiotics in IBS is rapidly growing. Our understanding of the possible physiologic mechanisms of improvement, particularly via alterations in immunomodulatory cytokines, represents the dawn of a new era in our approach to studying these therapies. We should be cautiously optimistic in our application of the current data. Most studies have small populations and a short length of treatment, especially given the waxing and waning nature of IBS. Trials of larger size and longer duration are needed to better clarify which probiotics work for which IBS symptom complex, as well as their mechanism of action and evidence for or against probiotics in patients with IBS remains elusive.

References

1. Young PE, Cash BD. Probiotic use in irritable bowel syndrome. *Current Gastroenterology Reports*. 2006;8:321-326.
2. Joint FAO/WHO Working Group Report on Drafting Guidelines for the Evaluation of Probiotics in Food. London, Ontario, Canada: May 1, 2002. Available at: http://www.who. int/foodsafety/fs_management/en/probiotic_guidelines.pdf. Accessed June 13, 2006.
3. Tsuchiya J, Barreto R, Okura R, et al. Single-blind follow-up study on the effectiveness of a symbiotic preparation in irritable bowel syndrome. *Chin J Dig Dis*. 2004;5(4):169-174.
4. Kim HJ, Vasquez-Roque MI, Camilleri M, et al. A randomized controlled trial of a probiotic combination VSL #3 and placebo in irritable bowel syndrome with bloating. *Neurogastroenterol Motil*. 2005;17(5):687-696.
5. Nobaek S, Johansson ML, Molin G, et al. Alteration in intestinal microflora is associated with reduction in abdominal bloating and pain in patients with irritable bowel syndrome. *Am J Gastroenterol*. 2000,95(5):1231-1238.
6. O'Mahony L, McCarthy J, Kelly P, et al. *Lactobacillus* and *bifidobacterium* in irritable bowel syndrome: symptom responses and relationship to cytokine profiles. *Gastroenterology*. 2005;128(3):541-551.
7. Niv E, Naftali T, Hallak R, Vaisman N. The efficacy of *Lactobacillus reuteri* ATCC 55730 in the treatment of patients with irritable bowel syndrome: a double blind, placebo-controlled, randomized study. *Clin Nutr*. 2005;24(6):925-931.

WHAT IS THE EVIDENCE FOR ANTIBIOTICS AS A THERAPY FOR IRRITABLE BOWEL SYNDROME?

Brian Mulhall, MD

The concept of augmenting the management of irritable bowel syndrome (IBS) with antibiotics is evolving, and many questions remain regarding this therapy relative to known and hypothesized IBS pathophysiology. The clinical evidence of small intestinal bacterial overgrowth (SIBO) as an important etiology of IBS continues to accumulate. Clinical symptoms of bacterial overgrowth and IBS are similar; however, a definitive cause-and-effect relationship remains unproven. It is unclear whether motility dysfunction causes bacterial overgrowth, or gas products of enteric bacteria affect intestinal motility in IBS.

Antibiotics, an emerging therapy for IBS, differ from the therapies typically used against the symptoms of IBS by targeting a putative pathogenic mechanism of the disorder, namely the hypothesis that SIBO might explain the physiologic hallmarks of altered gut motility, visceral hypersensitivity, abnormal brain-gut interaction, and immune activation seen in IBS.[1] Multiple lines of evidence support the putative role of bacteria in the development of IBS symptoms. Gas analysis is abnormal in 10% to 84% of IBS patients undergoing lactulose breath testing (Table 24-1).[2-7] Additionally, the distribution of inflammatory mediators and/or inflammatory cells has been shown to be disturbed in some patients with IBS. It is thought that SIBO may contribute too many of the clinical manifestations of IBS through bacterial fermentation and stimulation of a gut immune response, characterized by release of inflammatory mediators, such as interleukins and tumor necrosis factor-α, which may affect motility, secretion, and sensation. Bloating and gas, potentially arising from bacterial fermentation of dietary starch, are among the primary symptoms of IBS regardless of subtype (IBS-Constipation, IBS-Diarrhea, or IBS-Alternating). Postinfectious IBS, which occurs in 4% to 31% of individuals assessed up to 12 months after an episode of acute gastroenteritis, also supports an etiologic role of bacteria in IBS.

Table 24-1

Prevalence of Small Intestinal Bacterial Overgrowth in Irritable Bowel Syndrome Based on the Lactulose Breath Test

Lactulose Study	Number of Patients	Prevalence Percentage
Pimentel et al 2000	202	76
Nucera et al 2005	98	65
Pimentel et al 2003	111	84
Pimentel et al 2004	200	75
Walters and Vanner 2005	39	10
Noddin et al 2005	20	10

Results of clinical trials demonstrate that the reduction or elimination of SIBO with antibiotics can alleviate IBS symptoms.[2,4,8] The systemic antibiotic, neomycin, has been evaluated in two clinical studies.[4,8] In a double-blind, randomized, placebo-controlled study, neomycin dosed at 500 mg twice daily for 10 days was more effective than placebo at improving symptom scores among patients meeting Rome I criteria for IBS.[4] Additionally, a subanalysis of a double-blind, randomized, placebo-controlled trial demonstrated that treatment with neomycin improved global symptoms in individuals with constipation-predominant IBS compared with placebo ($P<.001$).[8]

The nonabsorbed (<0.4%), oral antibiotic rifaximin is the most thoroughly studied antibiotic for the treatment of IBS. Rifaximin appears to be well suited for the treatment of IBS because of its broad-spectrum bactericidal activity in vitro, its efficacy for SIBO in vivo, favorable tolerability profile, and lack of association with clinically relevant resistance or *Clostridium difficile* colitis. The efficacy of rifaximin in the treatment of IBS was evaluated in a randomized, double-blind, placebo-controlled, parallel-group study of 87 patients who met Rome I criteria for IBS.[9] These patients had not received oral antibiotics in the 3 months prior to the study and were not being treated with tegaserod or antidepressants. Patients received rifaximin at a dose of 400 mg 3 times daily or identical placebo 3 times daily for 10 days. At the end of treatment, more patients in the rifaximin group reported global improvement in IBS symptoms (37.7% vs 23.4%, $P<.05$), clinical response (ie, >50% improvement) (37.2% vs 15.9%, $P<.05$), and substantial improvement in diarrhea ($P<.05$) and bloating ($P=.06$). Treatment differences between rifaximin and placebo for the symptoms of constipation and abdominal pain were not statistically significant. Statistically significant improvement in IBS symptoms was observed with rifaximin over placebo during the 10-week follow-up period among 80 of the 87 patients who had at least one follow-up assessment. The maintenance of improvement during the 10-week follow-up period after a finite course of therapy suggests that chronic antibiotic treatment is not necessary for sustained clinical benefit, though larger studies of longer duration are needed to confirm this observation.

Long-term therapeutic benefits of rifaximin were also observed in two studies that assessed the effects of rifaximin on other functional GI symptoms.[10] In the Rifaximin in Abdominal Bloating and Flatulence Trial (RAFT), which involved 104 patients with functional GI symptoms (74 fulfilled Rome I criteria for IBS), the percentage of patients with global symptom relief was higher with rifaximin 400 mg twice daily than with placebo at the end of a 10-day course of therapy (41.3% vs 22.9%, $P=.03$). This difference persisted through the 30-day post-treatment observation period, with 28.6% of rifaximin-treated patients and 11.5% of placebo-treated patients reporting global symptom relief at the conclusion of this period ($P=.02$).

In another study, 34 patients with functional GI disorders received rifaximin 400 mg twice daily for 7 days or activated charcoal 300 mg twice daily for 7 days. Rifaximin, but not activated charcoal, reduced intestinal gas production (measured by hydrogen excretion) on the 1st and 10th days after completion of therapy compared with baseline values. Rifaximin also significantly reduced the number of flatus episodes, abdominal girth, and overall severity of symptoms on the 10th day after therapy completion compared with baseline values ($P<.05$). Numeric, but not statistically significant, reductions from baseline in bloating and abdominal pain were also observed on the 10th day after completion of therapy with rifaximin. With activated charcoal, no statistically significant effect was observed for any of these parameters.

Additional trials with antibiotics for IBS are eagerly awaited. Many questions remain regarding their use, however. To be a useful therapy for IBS, a non-life-threatening condition, a pharmacologic agent must be safe and well tolerated. Such an approach should also be cost effective and, ideally, provide long-lasting benefit. A short course of antibiotics is an attractive approach for IBS, but the utility and safety of repeated courses of antibiotics has not been well studied. The need for objective evidence of SIBO prior to therapy versus empiric therapy is also a hot topic without a clear answer. My current approach to using antibiotics in IBS is to treat patients with a prominent complaint of bloating with rifaximin, 800 mg 3 times daily for 10 days. I do not typically obtain lactulose breath tests prior to treatment and am comfortable treating empirically. Because this drug is not Food and Drug Administration approved for this indication, issues may arise regarding payment via third-party payers and can often be resolved through aggressive patient advocacy and discussion of the literature.

References

1. Lin HC. Small intestinal bacterial overgrowth: a framework for understanding irritable bowel syndrome. *JAMA*. 2004;292(7):852-858.
2. Pimentel M, Chow EJ, Lin HC. Eradication of small intestinal bacterial overgrowth reduces symptoms of irritable bowel syndrome. *Am J Gastroenterol*. 2000;95(12):3503-3506.
3. Nucera G, Gabrielli M, Lupascu A, et al. Abnormal breath tests to lactose, fructose and sorbitol in irritable bowel syndrome may be explained by small intestinal bacterial overgrowth. *Aliment Pharmacol Ther*. 2005;21(11):1391-1395.
4. Pimentel M, Chow EJ, Lin HC. Normalization of lactulose breath testing correlates with symptom improvement in irritable bowel syndrome: a double-blind, randomized, placebo-controlled study. *Am J Gastroenterol*. 2003;98:412-419.

5. Pimentel M, Wallace D, Hallegua D, et al. A link between irritable bowel syndrome and fibromyalgia may be related to findings on lactulose breath testing. *Ann Rheum Dis.* 2004;63(4):450-452.
6. Walters B, Vanner SJ. Detection of bacterial overgrowth in IBS using the lactulose H2 breath test: comparison with 14C-D-xylose and healthy controls. *Am J Gastroenterol.* 2005;100(7):1566-1570.
7. Noddin L, Callahan M, Lacy BE. Irritable bowel syndrome and functional dyspepsia: different diseases or a single disorder with different manifestations? *MedGenMed.* 2005;7(3):17.
8. Pimentel M, Chatterjee S, Chow EJ, Park S, Kong Y. Neomycin improves constipation-predominant irritable bowel syndrome in a fashion that is dependent on the presence of methane gas: subanalysis of a double-blind randomized controlled study. *Dig Dis Sci.* 2006;51(8):1297-1301.
9. Pimentel M, Park S, Kane SV. Rifaximin, a nonabsorbable, gut-selective antibiotic, improves the symptoms of irritable bowel syndrome: a randomized, double-blind, placebo-controlled study. *Ann Intern Med.* 2006;145(8):557-563.
10. Frissora CL, Cash BD. Review article: the role of antibiotics vs. conventional pharmacotherapy in treating symptoms of irritable bowel syndrome. *Aliment Pharmacol Ther.* 2007;25(11):1271-1281.

A PATIENT IN THE MIDST OF AN INFLAMMATORY BOWEL DISEASE FLARE ALSO WAS POSITIVE FOR CLOSTRIDIUM DIFFICILE. HOW OFTEN DOES THIS HAPPEN AND WHAT'S THE BEST WAY TO MANAGE THIS SCENARIO?

Brian Mulhall, MD

Clostridium difficile is the leading cause of hospital-acquired diarrhea. During the past decade, there has been an increase in the incidence of community-based *C. difficile* infections, and antibiotic resistance has increased. *C. difficile* can cause colitis itself, often referred to as pseudomembranous colitis, due to the plaques that adhere to the colonic mucosa (Figure 25-1). This infection can also occur in patients who have underlying inflammatory bowel diseases (IBD), like ulcerative colitis or Crohn's disease.[1] Patients with IBD are often treated with antibiotics and immunomodulators, which may increase the likelihood of infection with *C. difficile*. It appears that the incidence of *C. difficile* infection in patients with and without IBD is increasing.[1-3] One study has shown the incidence of *C. difficile* colitis in patients with a pre-existing diagnosis of IBS increased from 1.8% in 2004 to 4.6% in 2005 (*P*<.01).[1] Further, the proportion of IBD patients among all patients that presented with *C. difficile* infections doubled in that same time period (from 7% to 16%). Most of these cases developed in the outpatient setting, and more than half of these patients had been recently treated with an antibiotic. Another study showed that between 1998 and 2004, the rates of *C. difficile* infection doubled in patients with Crohn's disease and tripled in patients with ulcerative colitis.[2] These patients can be severely ill and upwards of 50% may require hospitalization. One in five may require colectomy.[1]

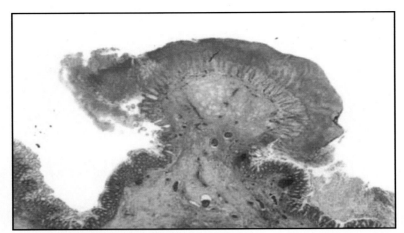

Figure 25-1. Photomicrograph of the colonic mucosa in a patient with ulcerative colitis and *C. difficile* colitis. Note the necrosis of the superficial crypts with a dense infiltrate of neutrophils and a plaque-like pseudomembrane of neutrophils, fibrin, and cellular debris covering the mucosal surface.

Chronic inflammation of the colon may be an important predisposing factor for infection. While small intestinal infections with *C. difficile* are uncommon, a recent case series described 6 patients who developed *C. difficile* enteritis after colectomy.[4] The increasing incidence of *C. difficile* infection in patients with IBD makes it difficult to ascertain if a patient with increasing diarrhea or abdominal pain is experiencing an IBD flare or a concomitant infection with *C. difficile*. Distinguishing between the two conditions is important due to the diametric differences in treatment. Although intravenous (IV) corticosteroids have been suggested as an option for severe refractory *C. difficile*, such an approach may be deleterious in patients with acute infection. In contrast, steroids and immunomodulators are considered the mainstays of therapy for IBD flares.

Stool study use to diagnose *C. difficile* infection in patients with IBD can produce mixed results.[5,6] Fecal leukocytes may be positive in both *C. difficile* infection and IBD, and the low sensitivity of the *C. difficile* toxin assay requires that at least 3 stool samples be collected, usually over several days, in order to feel relatively confident that an infection is not present. The classic endoscopic findings of pseudomembranes or fibrinopurulent plaques may not be seen in an IBD patient with concomitant *C. difficile* infection, so a high clinical suspicion is critical and early evaluation is important. Given the frequency of bowel movements in the setting of worsening IBD or a *C. difficile* infection, multiple stool samples may be sent in a single day. Given the possibility of poorer outcomes with *C. difficile* infection in IBD patients, arguments may need to be made for serial single-day sampling at institutions that have policies for only processing a single sample per day. If stool studies are unrevealing, flexible sigmoidoscopy or colonoscopy may be required, with biopsies of any inflamed mucosa. The pathologist should be alerted to the clinical suspicion of *C. difficile* infection so special tissue cultures can be performed, if required. If doubt remains or clinical suspicion for a superimposed infection with *C. difficile* is high, empiric antibiotic therapy (with metronidazole) may be warranted while the workup continues. In cases of fulminant colitis, where endoscopy may be contraindicated, *C. difficile* toxin assays are essential, and empiric therapy with appropriate antibiotics and IV corticosteroids is prudent.

References

1. Issa M, Vijayapal A, Graham MB, et al. Impact of *Clostridium difficile* on inflammatory bowel disease. *Clin Gastroenterol Hepatol.* 2007;5(3):345-351.
2. Rodemann JF, Dubberke ER, Reske KA, Seo da H, Stone CD. Incidence of *Clostridium difficile* infection in inflammatory bowel disease. *Clin Gastroenterol Hepatol.* 2007;5(3):339-344.
3. Pépin J, Valiquette L, Alary ME, et al. *Clostridium difficile*-associated diarrhea in a region of Quebec from 1991 to 2003: a changing pattern of disease severity. *CMAJ.* 2004;171(5):466-472.
4. Lundeen SJ, Otterson MF, Binion DG, Carman ET, Peppard WJ. *Clostridium difficile* enteritis: an early postoperative complication in inflammatory bowel disease patients after colectomy. *J Gastrointest Surg.* 2007;11(2):138-142.
5. Markowitz JE, Brown KA, Mamula P, Drott HR, Piccoli DA, Baldassano RN. Failure of single-toxin assays to detect *clostridium difficile* infection in pediatric inflammatory bowel disease. *Am J Gastroenterol.* 2001; 96(9):2688-2690.
6. Meyer AM, Ramzan NN, Loftus EV Jr, Heigh RI, Leighton JA. The diagnostic yield of stool pathogen studies during relapses of inflammatory bowel disease. *J Clin Gastroenterol.* 2004;38(9):772-775.

THE NURSING STAFF DOESN'T KNOW WHAT TO DO FOR A 72-HOUR STOOL COLLECTION AS PART OF A DIARRHEA WORKUP. WHAT DO I NEED TO TELL THEM TO GET THE ANSWERS I NEED?

Brian Mulhall, MD

When the cause of chronic diarrhea is elusive or there is a suspicion for malabsorption, a 72-hour stool collection may be warranted.[1] Many patients may report diarrhea, but it is important to realize that this term may be a subjective description of stool habits and may connote a variety of symptoms. Patients with 1 to 2 loose stools per day may report diarrhea as might patients who pass 3 to 4 formed stools per day. Recall that the medical definition of diarrhea is based on stool volume and requires more than 200 g of stool to be passed per day. A 72-hour stool collection serves as an objective quantification of fecal output and may help to clarify where further workup may be required.

There are some important practical issues in conducting a 72-hour stool study. Before embarking on this study, consider that several spot tests for steatorrhea are available that can obviate the need for a full 3-day collection. The Sudan III, the acid steatocrit, and a new technology (near infrared reflectance analysis) can have sensitivities as high as 90% to 100% in patients with clinically significant steatorrhea. The single sample approach makes these options attractive for outpatient evaluations or as a preliminary study before embarking on the 72-hour collection. While 72-hour stool collections may be done at home or in the hospital, admission promises to promote the most accurate results.[2] Patients and staff should be instructed to begin and end the collection at the same time 3 days apart.

The first bowel movement after waking on day 1 is generally considered the optimal starting point. Patients and staff should also be coached on how to collect the stool without contaminating the sample with urine. A standardized diet is also important. In order to be diagnostic of steatorrhea, a patient must consume at least 70 g to 120 g of fat in his or her diet each day of the study. If he or she consumes less fat than the prescribed amount, there is a risk of a false-negative result, and consultation with a dietician can be valuable to ensure adequate fat intake during the study. Additionally, the nursing staff needs to record the amount of actual meal consumption to ensure that the appropriate diet for the study was not underconsumed. All stool needs to be collected throughout the duration of the study. This is an imperative for an accurate result. Informing patients and staff that a missed stool could require reinitiation of the study may help with compliance. All collected stool should be refrigerated and delivered in total to the laboratory for assessment.

If there is concern for laxative abuse, the staff should be advised to ensure that the patient does not have access to laxatives during the admission. Depending upon the clinical scenario, stool should be tested for reducing substances, phenolphthalein, weight, volume, bacterial and viral culture, parasitologic examination, osmolality, electrolytes, fat content, meat fibers, and pH.

In summary, a 72-hour stool study can be invaluable in clarifying the diagnosis of chronic diarrhea and/or malabsorption. Ensuring adequate oral intake of fat and a complete collection of stool is paramount in obtaining an accurate result. If the patient has steatorrhea, then it may also be important to evaluate for endocrine insufficiency.

References

1. Schiller LR. Chronic diarrhea. *Gastroenterology.* 2004;127(1):287-293.
2. Schiller LR. Management of diarrhea in clinical practice: strategies for primary care physicians. *Rev Gastroenterol Disord.* 2007;7(suppl 3):S27-38.

I Want to Use Alosetron for a Woman With IBS-D. What Do I Need to Tell Her About the Risks and Outcomes Associated With Ischemic Colitis and This Medicine? What Is the Best Way to Document This Discussion?

Richard Saad, MD

Alosetron is a potent selective 5-HT$_3$ (serotonin) receptor antagonist. Its physiologic effects on the gastrointestinal tract include slowing colonic transit, decreasing visceral sensation, and increasing fluid absorption in the small intestine. Its efficacy in the treatment of women suffering from irritable bowel syndrome with diarrhea (IBS-D) has been proven in several high-quality randomized, placebo-controlled clinical trials.[1] Alosetron is superior to placebo in providing adequate relief of pain and discomfort, control of urgency, decreased stool frequency, and increased stool consistency.[1,2] Alosetron was initially approved in February 2000 for the treatment of women suffering from IBS-D. Due to post-marketing reports of severe constipation with complications such as fecal impaction, intestinal/ileus obstruction, toxic megacolon, and intestinal perforation as well as ischemic colitis, alosetron was withdrawn from the market in June 2000.

Largely due to public demand, alosetron was reintroduced in June 2002 for restricted use in women with severe IBS-D meeting specific indications. All of the following criteria must be met when considering the use of alosetron: 1) presence of IBS-D symptoms for a minimum of 6 months, 2) exclusion of anatomic and biochemical abnormalities of the gastrointestinal tract, and 3) lack of response to conventional therapy. In order to qualify as having "severe IBS-D," a woman has to report a least one of the following symptoms: 1) frequent and severe abdominal pain/discomfort, 2) frequent bowel urgency or fecal incontinence, or 3) disability or restriction in daily activities due to IBS symptoms. Contraindications to therapy were expanded to include a history of constipation, intestinal obstruction, stricture, toxic megacolon, gastrointestinal perforation, adhesions, ischemic colitis, impaired intestinal circulation, thrombophlebitis, hypercoagulable state, inflammatory bowel disease, diverticulitis, or severe liver impairment. A relative contraindication includes use in elderly (>65 years) women. In order to prescribe alosetron, a physician must be enrolled in a prescribing program sponsored by the makers of alosetron. Enrollment information can be easily accessed online at www.lotronex.com. Once registered, the physician will receive stickers that must be placed on all alosetron prescriptions.

Clinicians interested in prescribing alosetron should be familiar with the following information culled from clinical trial data and post-marketing surveillance. In clinical trials of the drug, constipation was most the common complaint reported in 29% of those taking 1 mg twice daily and in 11% of those taking 0.5 mg twice daily compared to 6% with placebo. Overall, 11% of patients discontinued therapy due to constipation, although only 4% discontinued therapy when taking 0.5 mg twice daily. Of the 11,874 patients receiving alosetron in these trials, there were 19 reports of ischemic colitis, yielding an incidence rate of 6.4 cases per 1000 patient-years.[3] Although 9 patients required hospitalization, all cases of ischemic colitis resolved without surgery or long-term sequelae. There were also 10 incidents of severe constipation with complications in these clinical trials yielding a rate of 3.3 cases per 1000 patient-years.[3] Of the 89 cases of reported ischemic colitis in post-marketing surveillance, 53 cases remained following adjudication with 36 requiring hospitalization, 3 requiring surgery, and no deaths.[3] There were also 5 cases of mesenteric ischemia in the initial post-marketing period, all requiring surgery, and one death. The association with alosetron in these cases remains unclear, and there have been no cases of mesenteric ischemia reported since the reintroduction of alosetron. Of the 108 cases of reported serious complications of constipation in post-marketing analysis, 31 remained following adjudication with 29 requiring hospitalization, 10 requiring surgery, and 2 deaths.[3] These results yielded a post-adjudication incidence of ischemic colitis to be 1.1 cases per 1000 patient-years and that of severe, complicated constipation to be 0.66 cases per 1000 patient-years.

Any patient choosing to pursue treatment with alosetron must be fully educated on the risks and benefits of the medication prior to receiving a prescription. Patients should receive and read a copy of the Alosetron Medication Guide. This 2-page document, developed by the manufacturer and approved by the Food and Drug Administration, is a mandatory part of prescribing alosetron. It is available from the manufacturer or online at www.lotronex.com. The document provides bulleted details regarding dosing, indications, contraindications, benefits, risks, and adverse effects of alosetron. The patient should be given an opportunity to ask questions after reading this document. Upon completion of these steps, the patient and physician must sign the Patient-Physician Agreement form, with one copy retained by the patient and the other copy retained in the patient's medical record. Initial dosing of alosetron is 0.5 mg twice daily, with an increase to 1 mg twice daily at 4 weeks if the starting dose does not adequately control IBS-D symptoms.

References

1. Cremonini F, Delgado-Aros S, Camilleri M. Efficacy of alosetron in irritable bowel syndrome: a meta-analysis of randomized controlled trials. *Neurogastroenterol Motil.* 2003;15(1):79-86.
2. Chey WD, Chey WY, Heath AT, et al. Long-term safety and efficacy of alosetron in women with severe diarrhea-predominant irritable bowel syndrome. *Am J Gastroenterol.* 2004;99(11):2195-2203.
3. Chang L, Chey WD, Harris L, Olden K, Surawicz C, Schoenfeld P. Incidence of ischemic colitis and serious complications of constipation among patients using alosetron: systematic review of clinical trials and post-marketing surveillance data. *Am J Gastroenterol.* 2006;101(5):1069-1079.

FOR PATIENTS WHO REPORT PERSISTENT DIARRHEA, WHAT IS CONSIDERED CHRONIC, WHEN DO I NEED TO BEGIN A WORKUP, AND WHAT DOES THAT WORKUP INVOLVE?

Richard Saad, MD

Diarrhea may be defined as a decrease in stool consistency (increased liquidity) or increase in stool frequency. Historically, it has been objectively defined as more than 3 daily bowel movements or the production of more than 200 g of stool in a 24-hour time period. Regardless of the criteria used, diarrhea is exceedingly common. The overwhelming majority of cases consist of acute diarrhea. They are typically self-limited, resolving over a period of several days and rarely requiring more than supportive care. However, the scenario changes significantly with chronic diarrhea due to the complexity of the potential causes, diagnostic evaluation, and treatment. It is therefore essential to recognize the difference between an acute diarrhea and that of a chronic diarrhea. Symptoms persisting for more than 4 weeks have been arbitrarily defined as chronic diarrhea.[1] A presentation of chronic diarrhea always warrants further investigation. At a minimum, this should consist of a detailed history, physical examination, routine laboratory studies, and stool analysis. Further directed testing is then pursued based on findings from this initial evaluation.

A careful and comprehensive history is essential as it can frequently help to distinguish an organic diarrhea from that of a functional diarrhea. The American Gastroenterological Association and British Society of Gastroenterology have detailed the essential elements of a history in a patient with chronic diarrhea.[2,3] These should include delineation of the following: 1) onset of diarrhea (congenital, sudden, or gradual); 2) pattern of diarrhea (nocturnal, continuous, or intermittent symptoms); 3) duration of symptoms; 4) epidemiologic factors (recent travel, exposure to contaminated food or water, or family history of gastrointestinal illness); 5) stool characteristics (volume and description of watery, bloody, or fatty); 6) presence of fecal incontinence; 7) presence of abdominal pain or weight loss; 8) mitigating, aggravating, and alleviating features (food, stress, drugs); 9) detailed medication history; 10) coexistent systemic diseases (thyroid dysfunction, diabetes mellitus, collagen-vascular diseases, cancer, acquired immunodeficiency syndrome, or pancreatic disease); 11) previous surgery or radiation therapy; 12) alcohol history; 13) recent antibiotic use or history of *Clostridium difficile* infection; 14) review of previous evaluations; and 15) history of laxative use, eating disorders, malingering, or secondary gains. The information gathered here may help to distinguish irritable bowel syndrome, fecal incontinence, iatrogenic, or factitious diarrhea from organic chronic diarrhea.

While typically less revealing than the history, a physical examination is also an essential component of the initial evaluation.[2] The nutritional and fluid status should be assessed, and one should evaluate for the presence of flushing, skin rashes, oral ulcers, thyroid enlargement, joint inflammation, heart murmur, wheezing, abdominal masses, hepatomegaly, ascites, peripheral edema, sphincter incompetence, perianal abscess, or fistula.

Initial laboratory testing should include minimal screening serologic and stool studies.[1,3] Blood work should consist of a complete blood count, erythrocyte sedimentation rate, basic serum electrolytes, serum albumin and protein, liver panel, and thyroid stimulating hormone level. Serologic testing for celiac disease (serum IgA with tissue transglutaminase, antiendomysial, or antigliadin antibodies) should also be considered, particularly in patients of Northern European ancestry and those with diabetes mellitus, osteoporosis, or family history of celiac disease. Stool studies should include hemoccult testing at a minimum. Additional stool testing for *Clostridium difficile* toxin, *Giardia lamblia* antigen, ova and parasites, fecal fat, stool electrolytes, and pH should be based on the history and physical exam. If malabsorption is suspected, a 72-hour stool collection may be useful.

Following this initial evaluation, the presence of any alarm features (Table 28-1) or clinical suspicion of an organic cause for the diarrhea should mandate further structural evaluation. Colonoscopy with ileoscopy and biopsy should be the initial structural studies performed. A recent retrospective chart review revealed a histologic diagnosis in 31% of patients with chronic diarrhea following colonoscopy with biopsy.[4] Further endoscopic evaluation may also include upper endoscopy with biopsy in the event that celiac serologic testing is positive, associated upper gastrointestinal symptoms exist, or an upper gastrointestinal structural etiology is suspected.

Additional testing or empiric treatment trials would be based on symptoms or findings suggesting a specific cause. Computed tomography, small bowel radiography, or small endoscopy should be considered in a patient with alarm features and unrevealing colonoscopy/EGD. Breath testing for bacterial overgrowth or lactase deficiency may be pursued if there is associated bloating and abdominal pain with the diarrhea. Empiric treatment for presumed post-cholecystectomy or small bowel bacterial overgrowth may also be considered. Further testing for pancreatic insufficiency may be pursued if there is evidence of fat malabsorption or history/radiography suggestive of pancreatic disease. Serologic testing for neuroendocrine tumors and other hormone-secreting tumors should be considered at this point, particularly in secretory diarrhea that is difficult to treat. These are rare causes of chronic diarrhea and frequently have associated syndromes.

Table 28-1

Alarm Features

Historical

- Age >50 years
- Rectal bleeding or hematochezia
- Unintentional weight loss
- Family history of GI malignancy
- Severe (unrelenting or prolonged) diarrhea
- Severe (unrelenting or prolonged) abdominal pain
- Fever
- Travel to endemic area
- Nocturnal symptoms

Physical Exam

- Arthritis
- Skin abnormalities
- Lymphadenopathy
- Abdominal mass
- Hepatomegaly/splenomegaly
- Mucosal ulcers
- Perianal fistula or abscess

Laboratory

- Anemia
- Elevated erythrocyte sedimentation rate
- Positive stool occult blood test

In summary, diarrheal symptoms persisting for more than 4 weeks constitute a diagnosis of chronic diarrhea. Chronic diarrhea warrants further evaluation with the goal of distinguishing an organic cause from that of nonorganic cause. The history and physical exam, basic laboratory and stool studies, and endoscopy will permit determination of the diagnosis in most cases.

References

1. Fine KD, Schiller LR. AGA technical review on the evaluation and management of chronic diarrhea. *Gastroenterology.* 1999;116(6):1464-1486.
2. American Gastroenterological Association medical position statement: guidelines for the evaluation and management of chronic diarrhea. *Gastroenterology.* 1999;116(6):1461-1463.
3. Thomas PD, Forbes A, Green J, et al. Guidelines for the investigation of chronic diarrhoea, 2nd edition. *Gut.* 2003;52(suppl 5):v1-15.
4. Shah RJ, Fenoglio-Preiser C, Bleau BL, Giannella RA. Usefulness of colonoscopy with biopsy in the evaluation of patients with chronic diarrhea. *Am J Gastroenterol.* 2001;96(4):1091-1095.

MY PATIENT WITH COLLAGENOUS COLITIS DEVELOPED A BLACK TONGUE WITH BISMUTH. WHAT OTHER THERAPEUTIC OPTIONS DO I HAVE?

Richard Saad, MD

Collagenous colitis represents one of the two major forms of microscopic colitis. This is an idiopathic, chronic condition marked by nonbloody, watery diarrhea and characteristic histologic abnormalities on mucosal biopsy. Associated symptoms may include occasional fecal incontinence, abdominal cramping, nausea, weight loss, and abdominal distention. Endoscopy and radiographic studies are normal, and laboratory studies are generally unremarkable as well. The mucosal abnormalities of collagenous colitis include a thickened linear subepithelial collagen layer and frequently a mononuclear (lymphocytes, plasma cell, and/or macrophages) cellular infiltrate with epithelial cell damage. Collagenous colitis has an incidence of 4 to 6 per 100,000 people. It occurs more commonly in women and the elderly, with a median age at onset of 65 years, although it has been diagnosed in all ages, including children. There are no known long-term colonic complications of this condition. Although symptoms may wax and wane, the primary objective of treatment is the effective control of the diarrhea and any accompanying lower abdominal symptoms. A variety of treatments exist to include antidiarrheals, fiber supplementation, binding agents, 5-aminosalicylates, antibiotics, immunosuppressants, antisecretory agents, and surgery. There are limited controlled studies assessing these treatment strategies as their use is largely based on anecdotal evidence and that of small, poorly controlled trials. Thus, the choice of treatment is based on a careful balance of symptom severity with that of the risks of therapy.

Bismuth subsalicylate is frequently used as a first-line agent in the treatment of collagenous colitis given its low expense, ease of administration, and relatively low risk of side effects. Its effectiveness is largely based on a single small trial only published in abstract form.[1] In this study, nine 262 mg tablets of bismuth subsalicylate taken daily in 3 divided doses for 8 weeks were compared to placebo in patients with collagenous colitis. Those receiving bismuth had clinical improvement, and 6 of 7 also had histologic improvement. However, bismuth subsalicylate is associated with a number of adverse effects that have limited its availability in a number of countries. The more common side effects include darkening of the stool, skin, and tongue. The grayish-black tongue discoloration with bismuth subsalicylate is due to formation of bismuth sulfide and is harmless, although unsightly. Tinnitus has been reported as a result of salicylate absorption. A rare but severe complication is that of bismuth-related encephalopathy, which has occurred more commonly with bismuth compounds other than bismuth subsalicylate. Other infrequent but observed side effects from bismuth include rash, constipation, diarrhea, nausea, and vomiting.

In the event of treatment failure with bismuth subsalicylate, other relatively safe and reasonably inexpensive treatment strategies include loperamide, cholestyramine, sulfasalazine, or 5-aminosalicylic acid.[2] Although their effectiveness has only been reported in case reports and uncontrolled trials, they are frequently used in clinical practice. Boswellia serrata extract was studied in a single placebo-controlled trial involving 31 patients. A 6-week trial of therapy consisting of three 400-mg capsules daily only demonstrated a trend toward superiority over that of placebo in achieving clinical improvement. A number of probiotics have also been studied with some promising results, and antibiotics such as metronidazole and erythromycin have been reported to be effective in uncontrolled trials.

Budesonide, a glucocorticoid steroid with a high first-pass metabolism, is the best studied short-term treatment strategy for patients with collagenous colitis.[3] Three randomized controlled trials involving a total of 93 patients demonstrated the superiority of budesonide over placebo in the treatment of diarrhea, improvement in quality of life, and resolution of mucosal abnormalities. In these studies, a daily dose of 9 mg of budesonide was used for a period of 6 to 8 weeks. A pooled analysis revealed a number needed to treat of 2 to achieve a clinical response to budesonide.[2] However, the relapse rate upon discontinuation of budesonide was significant, occurring in 60% to 80% of patients within 2 weeks. An unproven strategy to prevent relapse may include the use of a low (3 mg to 6 mg) maintenance dose of budesonide. However, there is potential for the same adverse effects of long-term corticosteroid use (hyperglycemia, weight gain, osteoporosis, cataracts).

In the event of treatment failure with the previously described agents, more potent immunosuppressants such as prednisone, azathioprine, or methotrexate should be considered.[3] Only prednisone (50 mg daily dose) has been studied in a small placebo-controlled trial involving 11 patients with collagenous colitis. This study was limited by a short treatment period (2 weeks) and a lack of clear superiority of prednisone over placebo. The use of azathioprine and methotrexate remain unproven. Given the significant risk of adverse effects with use of these agents, they should be reserved for severely symptomatic patients who have failed prednisone. Surgical procedures include colectomy, sigmoidostomy, and ileostomy and should be considered in the rare circumstance of disease that is refractory to all forms of medical therapy.

In summary, there are multiple treatment alternatives for collagenous colitis, although limited data exist on their effectiveness. Given the generally benign course of collagenous colitis, it is important to carefully weigh the benefits with the risks and costs of the therapy chosen.

References

1. Fine KD, Ogunji F, Lee E, Lafon G, Tanzi M. Randomized, double blind, placebo-controlled trial of bismuth subsalicylate for microscopic colitis [abstract]. *Gastroenterology.* 1999;116:A880.
2. Chande N, McDonald JW, MacDonald JK. Interventions for treating collagenous colitis. *Cochrane Database Syst Rev.* 2006;18(4):CD003575.
3. Nyhlin N, Bohr J, Eriksson S, Tysk C. Systematic review: microscopic colitis. *Aliment Pharmacol Ther.* 2006;23(11):1525-1534.

SECTION IV

PERIANAL DISORDERS

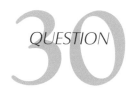

WHAT ARE THE TREATMENT OPTIONS FOR A PATIENT WITH METASTATIC COLON CANCER WHO HAS A MALIGNANT SIGMOID STRICTURE?

Brooks D. Cash, MD, FACP, FACG

Malignant colonic obstruction is the most common reason for emergent large bowel surgery, accounting for up to 85% of such cases. Patients with colorectal cancer who present with obstruction have a 5-year survival rate of less than 29%.[1] Approximately 15% to 30% of patients with colorectal cancer present with colonic obstruction, and historically the management of these patients involved creation of a diverting colostomy. This management schema has several drawbacks. Patients with malignant colonic obstructions cannot undergo a 1-stage operative tumor resection and re-anastamosis of the large bowel because stool present in the colonic segments proximal to the obstruction leads to breakdown of the anastamosis. While re-anastamosis is often one of the goals in the management of such patients, up to 40% never undergo successful stoma reversal.[2] Additionally, patients presenting with malignant colonic obstruction tend to be acutely ill, and the mortality rates associated with surgery for large bowel obstruction are relatively high, ranging from 8.8% to 27% in several series. Restoring bowel continuity and preoperative decompression offers several advantages. It allows clinical stabilization of the patient and colonic preparation so that a resection can be performed in a 1-stage fashion, thus avoiding creation of a colostomy. For some patients, restoring bowel continuity nonsurgically provides a window during which time they can undergo adjuvant or neo-adjuvant therapies as well. For another group of patients, nonoperative restoration of bowel continuity may be used as a palliative measure. At least 70% of colonic obstructions from colon cancer occur in the left side of the colon and thus may be amenable to restoration of continuity via the placement of stents.

Self-expandable metal stents (SEMS) are gaining increasing use in the management of patients with malignant intestinal strictures.[3] SEMS come in a variety of metallic alloys, shapes, and sizes, varying by manufacturer and intended uses of the stent.[4] Colonic SEMS have luminal diameters of 20 mm to 30 mm and work by exerting radial pressure to the colon wall, thus maintaining patency. Once deployed across the stricture, the stent becomes embedded within tumor and surrounding tissue through pressure necrosis. It also becomes deeply seated in colonic tissue on both the proximal and distal margins of the tumor, providing anchoring sites so that stent migration does not occur. Covered stents (frequently used in other parts of the gastrointestinal tract) are not typically used for malignant colon strictures because the covering can prevent the aforementioned anchoring and can increase the risk of stent migration. SEMS may be placed either endoscopically or through interventional radiology. Once placed, SEMS can affect image quality of both computed tomography and magnetic resonance imaging (MRI), depending on shape, composition, and, in the case of MRI, orientation to the magnetic field.

Much of the evidence supporting the use of SEMS compared to other management techniques for patients with malignant colonic obstructions is derived from case reports and clinical series. Sebastian and colleagues reported the results of a pooled analysis of 54 reports involving nearly 1200 patients.[5] In this review, two-thirds of patients underwent SEMS placement for definitive palliation while the other third underwent placement as a bridge to subsequent single stage resection. Most patients in this analysis had strictures related to colorectal cancer but 10% had strictures related to extrinsic compression from noncolonic malignancies and nearly two-thirds of the stents were placed endoscopically with fluoroscopic guidance. Technical success was achieved with the first attempt at SEMS placement in more than 93% of patients. Interestingly, the failure rate for rectosigmoid strictures was 5.8% while that for descending colon and more proximal strictures was 14.5% and 15.4%, respectively. Failure rates were slightly, but not significantly, higher for stents placed without endoscopic assistance. Strictures from extrinsic colonic compression were more likely than those from intrinsic colon tumors to defy successful SEMS placement (22% vs 6.5%). Complications included perforation in 3.8% (most often from stent wires or during balloon dilation), stent migration in 11.8%, and reobstruction in 7.3%. All but one of the perforations occurred at the rectosigmoid junction. Predilation did not appear to positively impact the success rate of SEMS placement, but was significantly associated with perforation risk. Most perforations required emergent surgery and were thought to play an important role in the deaths of 5 out of the 7 patients who expired. While the technical success of SEMS placement was quite high in this review, the results achieved with SEMS as a bridge to surgery were less impressive, preventing stoma creation in 71% of patients. There were a variety of causes for this result, most importantly the undetected presence of local tumor extension discovered at surgery and inadequate bowel preparation, even after stent placement. However, even with these limitations, SEMS placement appears to have both clinical and economic benefits compared to emergent surgery and stoma formation in the palliative and therapeutic arenas.

Education of the patient is also an important aspect of the successful placement of an SEMS. Many patients who undergo successful SEMS deployment continue to have some form of bowel dysfunction.[4] While this may be preferable to the costs associated with emergent surgery, patients should be carefully counseled regarding the possible risks and probable outcomes of SEMS placement. After successful placement and decompression, patients may resume oral intake and, in the case of patients who undergo SEMS for palliation, should be encouraged to consume a low-residue diet. It is also advisable to prescribe stool softeners or laxatives to maintain a soft or semi-solid stool to reduce the risk of stent migration in these patients. If tumor ingrowth occurs, many patients can be successfully treated with repeat stent placement or another palliative therapy such as argon-beam plasma coagulation or laser therapy directed at reducing intraluminal tumor burden.

References

1. Tekkis PP, Kinsman R, Thompson MR, et al. The Association of Coloproctology of Great Britain and Ireland study of large bowel obstruction caused by colorectal cancer. *Ann Surg.* 2004;240(1):76-81.
2. Deans GT, Krukowski ZH, Irwin ST. Malignant obstruction of the left colon. *Br J Surg.* 1994;81(9):1270-1276.
3. Mauro MA, Koehler RE, Baron TH. Advances in gastrointestinal intervention: the treatment of gastroduodenal and colorectal obstructions with metallic stents. *Radiology.* 2000;215(3):659-669.
4. Baron TH, Kozarek RA. Endoscopic stenting of colonic tumors. *Best Pract Res Clin Gastroenterol.* 2004;18(1):209-229.
5. Sebastian S, Johnston S, Geoghegan T, et al. Pooled analysis of the efficacy and safety of self-expanding metal stenting in malignant colorectal obstruction. *Am J Gastroenterol.* 2004;99(10):2051-2057.

WHAT SHOULD I BE DOING WITH MY PATIENTS WHO HAVE ANAL FISSURES?

Brian E. Lacy, MD, PhD

Anal fissures are tears or splits in the anal canal inferior to the dentate line. Fissures are a common problem, affecting up to 10% of the population. Men and women are equally susceptible; children and geriatric patients are less likely to be affected than younger and middle-aged adults. Many fissures are small and heal spontaneously before patients can seek medical advice. For treatment purposes, fissures may be categorized into acute (up to 6 weeks in duration) or chronic.

Anal fissures are characterized by pain and bleeding. Evacuation of stool generally produces severe anal pain, which may last for several hours afterwards. Small amounts of bright red blood may coat the stool or be found on the tissue paper. The pain can be so severe in some patients that they fear having a bowel movement.

Traditional teaching holds that straining and passing rocky, hard stool causes a tear in the anal canal. However, most patients with fissures are not constipated and many actually suffer from diarrhea. Most patients cannot recall an episode of acute constipation just prior to the development of a fissure. More recent studies have demonstrated that patients with fissures often have reduced blood flow to the anal canal (branches of the inferior rectal artery), especially in the posterior midline. In addition, anal canal pressures are elevated in patients with both chronic and acute anal fissures. The combination of elevated anal canal pressures with poor perfusion may produce localized ischemia, leading to the development of an ulcer that could tear with even minimal straining or trauma. Once a fissure develops, spasm of the internal anal sphincter can pull the wound edges further apart, preventing or delaying healing, leading to chronicity.[1]

The clinical history of anal pain after defecation in conjunction with episodic rectal bleeding is pathognomonic of an anal fissure. However, other disorders that must be included in the differential diagnosis are prolapsed hemorrhoids, a fissure associated with inflammatory bowel disease, and infectious disorders of the perianal area (syphilis, gonorrhea, herpes, HIV, tuberculosis). Some patients may also have symptoms of burning and itching, secondary to inflammation or persistent mucus or moisture at the site of the fissure. Physical examination begins with careful inspection of the perianal region, which can be difficult because the anal sphincter may be in spasm. However, it is critical that good exposure of the perianal region be obtained. An internal rectal examination is often impossible in patients with a fissure due to severe pain. A complete rectal examination often has to be performed under anesthesia.

The majority of fissures (90%) develop in the posterior midline; a skin tag (a "sentinel" tag or pile) is often seen at the inferior edge, while a hypertrophied papilla is often seen at the superior edge. Most fissures are fusiform or pear-shaped. Acute fissures characteristically have sharp edges, while chronic fissures have indurated edges and the horizontal fibers of the internal anal sphincter muscle may be seen. Of note, fissures associated with Crohn's disease are typically located in the lateral position.

In a young patient (<40 years of age) with characteristic symptoms and an anal fissure identified on rectal examination, treatment can be initiated without any diagnostic testing. Patients older than 50 years can be treated empirically; however, a screening colonoscopy is warranted if not previously performed. Younger patients who fail to respond to therapy, and those older than 40 with persistent symptoms of pain and bleeding despite appropriate therapy, should undergo flexible sigmoidoscopy to ensure that a second problem is not contributing to the patient's persistent symptoms.

Treatment begins by ensuring that patients have adequate fiber in their diets (25 to 30 g per day). Several placebo-controlled studies have demonstrated that treating anal fissure patients with fiber improves the rate and extent of wound healing.[1] Sitz baths keep the perianal area clean and help relax the anal sphincter. Topical anesthetics (eg, lidocaine) improve pain but do not improve healing. Topical nitroglycerin (0.2% to 0.3% ointment) applied twice daily for 4 to 6 weeks improves healing in a significant number of patients. Topical nitrates relax smooth muscle, allow wound edges to more closely appose, and improve blood flow to the anoderm, with the end result of fissure healing. Unfortunately, nitrates commonly produce side effects of headaches (up to 70% of patients), hypotension, and nausea, thus limiting their usefulness. Topical calcium channel blockers (eg, diltiazem) also produce smooth muscle relaxation and are less likely to cause the side effects noted with nitrates. A number of studies have demonstrated that botulinum toxin injection leads to improved wound healing.[2] Botulinum toxin works by inhibiting the release of acetylcholine. This causes the smooth muscle fibers to relax, enabling the wound edges to appose and heal. Injection of 20 to 40 units around the fissure can be safely accomplished in the office using a 25G needle. Botulinum toxin has been shown to be more effective than nitroglycerin in several head-to-head comparisons, and side effects are uncommon.

If medical treatments fail, some surgeons employ sequential anal dilation. This is thought to produce a small localized tear of the internal anal sphincter, thus promoting relaxation and healing of the fissure. However, this has been shown to be much less effective than true surgical sphincterotomy and may only improve pain due to the use of the anesthetic jelly used to coat the dilator. Lateral sphincterotomy is now considered to be the surgical treatment of choice, with healing rates of 90% to 95%.[3] It can be performed in a same-day surgery setting using topical anesthesia or under general anesthesia. Division of the anal sphincter causes the internal anal sphincter to relax and allows the wound edges to appose and heal. The most significant complication is incontinence, which can occur in up to 30% of patients. Chronic anal fissures are more likely to require, and to respond to, surgery as opposed to medical therapy.

References

1. Lund JN, Scholefield JH. Aetiology and treatment of anal fissure. *Br J Surg.* 1996;83(10):1335-1344.
2. Brisinda G, Maria G, Bentivoglio AR, et al. A comparison of injections of botulinum toxin and topical nitroglycerin ointment for the treatment of chronic anal fissure. *N Engl J Med.* 1999;341(2):65-69.
3. Richard CS, Gregoire R, Plewes EA, et al. Internal sphincterotomy is superior to topical nitroglycerin in the treatment of chronic anal fissure. *Dis Colon Rectum.* 2000;43(8):1048-1058.

WHAT IS PRURITUS ANI AND HOW IS IT MANAGED?

Brian E. Lacy, MD, PhD

Pruritus ani is a frustrating condition frequently seen by primary care providers, gastroenterologists, and colorectal surgeons. Although the exact prevalence is unknown, estimates are that it affects up to 5% of the US population, including all ages and both genders. Several studies have shown a male predominance, although the reasons for this are not known. Pruritus is not a single, specific disease, but rather the end result of any of a number of different pathophysiologic processes. As illustrated in Table 32-1, the differential diagnosis is quite broad.[1]

Patients with pruritus ani complain of itching, burning, or stinging in the perianal area. Symptoms may resolve spontaneously, and thus most patients who seek medical advice generally have chronic symptoms and likely have failed simple over-the-counter remedies. Symptoms are not relieved by having a bowel movement, and pruritus is not associated with bleeding. Symptoms are often worse at night, when patients are less distracted.

Pruritus ani essentially represents a localized response to irritation or inflammation, which may be limited to the superficial layers of the perianal area or involve deeper layers as well.[2] For example, rectal prolapse leads to excessive deposition of mucus on the perianal mucosa, which can irritate the skin, leading to macerated tissue. Alternatively, excess mucus may predispose the patient to develop candidiasis (*Candida albicans*), leading to chronic symptoms of burning and itching. Skin tags and fissures may interfere with proper hygiene, which can then set up a localized inflammatory response. Although the mechanism is unknown, some patients report that eliminating caffeine, cola, beer, tomatoes, chocolate, and tea improve symptoms. Less commonly, infiltrative processes, including anal malignancies, can produce symptoms of pruritus. No matter which process is initially involved, irritation causes the patient to itch or scratch the affected area, further exacerbating a localized inflammatory response. Further itching then ensues, and a vicious cycle of itch, scratch, itch is perpetuated. Finally, many patients with persistent symptoms feel as if they cannot keep

Table 32-1
Etiology of Pruritus Ani

Topical Irritants

- Soaps
- Deodorants
- Perfumes
- Dry cleaning solutions
- Allergies to dyes, fabric softeners
- Tight-fitting clothes (lack of air circulation, pressure)

Mechanical Factors

- Fissures
- Fistula
- Abscess
- Fecal incontinence
- Hemorrhoids
- Prolapse

Infections

- Candida
- Herpes simplex
- *Papillomavirus* (condyloma acuminata)
- *Staphylococcus aureus*
- *Corynebacterium* (erythrasma)
- Pinworms
- Scabies
- Syphilis
- Gonorrhea
- HIV

Dermatologic Disorders

- Psoriasis
- Seborrhea
- Lichen planus
- Lichen sclerosis
- Atopic dermatitis

Systemic Disorders

- Diabetes
- Lymphoma
- Aplastic anemia

Malignancies

- Bowen's disease
- Extramammary Paget's
- Squamous cell carcinoma

Miscellaneous

- Sensitivities to foods (tomatoes, citrus, beer, coffee, tea, cola)
- Medications (mineral oil, quinidine, colchicine)

the perianal area clean. This leads to excessive cleansing of the perianal area, which can further irritate the inflamed area.

The differential diagnosis for pruritus is broad and includes topical irritants, infections, dermatologic disorders, mechanical factors, systemic disorders, and malignancies (see Table 32-1). A good history is essential, and the patient should be questioned about excessive wiping or cleansing, especially with fragrant soaps. If the patient is diabetic, serum glucose control should be assessed. Physical examination of the perianal area reveals reddened, irritated skin in the acute setting. Scratch marks may be present. Fissures and skin tags should be identified, while a growth or raised lesion will be obvious. During the rectal examination, the patient should be asked to strain to determine if prolapse occurs. Patients with chronic symptoms may develop thick, whitened skin in this area consistent with lichenification. Contrary to current popular opinion, pinworms (*Enterobius vermicularis*) are an unlikely cause of pruritus in the United States. In the absence of warning signs (unintentional weight loss, anemia, rectal bleeding, family history of colorectal cancer), no other evaluation is required during the initial visit.

Educating the patient is paramount to resolving pruritus ani, because patients need to understand that persistent scratching and itching only further irritates the area and sets up a cycle of recurrent inflammation. Antihistamines, especially when used at night, can reduce nocturnal itching.[3] If diarrhea is thought to be a precipitating factor, this needs to be treated. Dietary modifications can be employed, although no controlled trials are available to guide either the patient or the practitioner. Sitz baths can be used to keep the area clean, and only fragrance-free soaps should be used. The patient should be counseled to avoid excessive wiping and cleansing. Some patients find that witch hazel pads can improve hygiene and minimize irritation. The area should be kept dry at all times. Some patients use a hair dryer to dry the perianal area after a shower or bath. Hydrocortisone cream (1%) can be used during the phase of treatment, but should not be used longer than 2 weeks.

References

1. Bowyer A, McColl I. A study of 200 patients with pruritus ani. *Pro R Soc Med.* 1970;63(suppl):96-98.
2. Friend WG. The cause of idiopathic pruritus ani. *Dis Colon Rectum.* 1977;20:40-42.
3. Fazio VW, Tjandra JJ. The management of perianal diseases. *Adv Surg.* 1996;29:59-78.

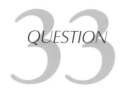

WHAT IS PROCTALGIA FUGAX AND HOW IS IT MANAGED?

Brian E. Lacy, MD, PhD

Proctalgia fugax (fugax-fleeting) is characterized by brief episodes of rectal pain. Although a common problem, information regarding this disorder is limited because the published medical literature consists mostly of anecdotal reports and small case series. Several prospective studies, however, have determined that the prevalence of proctalgia ranges from 3% to 14%.[1] Proctalgia occurs worldwide and affects men and women of all races and socioeconomic status, although there appears to be a slight female predominance.

Rectal pain is the defining characteristic of proctalgia.[2] Patients generally have fairly stereotypical episodes, although there is great variability in symptoms among patients. Proctalgia occurs unpredictably and without warning. Patients may describe the pain as sharp, stabbing, twisting, cramping, or lancinating in nature. Although patients often vividly remember nocturnal episodes because they cause sudden awakening, proctalgia can occur just as frequently during the day as well. The pain generally remains localized within the rectum, although occasionally the pain may radiate into the gluteal or perineal region. Episodes are generally brief in nature, ranging from seconds up to 30 minutes, with each painful episode resolving spontaneously. The exceptional patient may have an episode that lasts for days. Most patients have several episodes per year; it is the rare patient who has 2 or more episodes per month.

The pathophysiology of proctalgia is unknown, although it likely represents a spastic condition of the smooth muscle of the anal canal.[3] There is a limited amount of data to support spasm of the rectosigmoid as a cause, while some clinicians and researchers believe that proctalgia develops due to spasm of the levator ani muscles (primarily the pubococcygeus). Physiologic studies using anorectal manometry and endoanal ultrasound have shown that proctalgia patients are similar to healthy controls during pain-free episodes, although one study demonstrated that anal canal resting pressures were higher in patients with proctalgia than normal volunteers. One study found that, during episodes of pain, patients with proctalgia have increased anal canal pressures and an increase in the frequency of slow waves in the anal canal.[3] Patients frequently ask about precipitating factors, although no clear-cut precipitating event has been identified. Some patients report that straining at stool, stress, or intercourse may provoke an attack. Contrary to what has been written in many textbooks, proctalgia is not more likely to occur in patients with irritable bowel syndrome.

The diagnosis of proctalgia fugax can be made based on the clinical history.[2] Clinically, the pain of proctalgia is different than the persistent, dull ache associated with levator ani syndrome, or the fullness and pressure that may accompany hemorrhoidal prolapse. Fissure pain is usually more severe, longer lasting, and associated with bleeding.

A careful examination of the perianal region is imperative. Fissures, thrombosed hemorrhoids, masses, prolapse, and lichenification associated with chronic pruritus ani can all be quickly identified. Sensation can be quickly assessed, as can tone and strength of the external anal sphincter. Internal examination can identify a large rectocele, prolapse, or the taut muscle associated with levator ani syndrome (nearly always on the patient's left side). Although the history is diagnostic, patients are frequently worried about cancer because of the unpredictable and fleeting nature of the pain. In the current medico-legal climate, flexible sigmoidoscopy with careful retroflexion in the rectum should be performed.

Treating patients with proctalgia can be difficult, because symptoms have usually completely resolved by the time the patient can initiate medical therapy. In addition, because the majority of patients have very infrequent episodes, most clinicians are reticent to treat a patient with a daily medication in order to prevent a single, brief monthly episode. After carefully explaining the nature of the condition to the patient and reassuring him or her that it is a benign disorder, conservative therapy is generally the best recommendation. A warm sitz bath or even a warm water enema at the start of the attack can be very useful. Longer lasting episodes can be treated with short-acting benzodiazepines, smooth muscle antispasmodics (ie, sublingual hyoscyamine), sublingual nitroglycerin, or topical (perianal) nitroglycerin. One prospective, double-blind study demonstrated that an inhaled beta-agonist, salbuterol, shorted the length of each episode. Patients with frequent episodes may benefit from the use of a calcium channel blocker, long-acting nitrates, or even botulinum toxin injection of the anal canal. Some patients and physicians have resorted to myotomy of the anal canal as a last resort; however, that is generally not necessary, even in the most severe patients.

References

1. Drossman DA, Li Z, Andruzzi E, et al. US householder survey of functional gastrointestinal disorders. Prevalence, sociodemography, and health impact. *Dig Dis Sci*. 1993;38(9):1569-1580.
2. de Parades V, Etienney I, Bauer P, et al. Proctalgia fugax: demographic and clinical characteristics. What every doctor should know from a prospective study of 54 patients. *Dis Colon Rectum*. 2007;50(6):893-898.
3. Eckardt VF, Dodt O, Kanzler G, Bernhard G. Anorectal function and morphology in patients with sporadic proctalgia fugax. *Dis Colon Rectum*. 1996;39(7):755-762.

WHAT TYPES OF PROCEDURES AND THERAPIES CAN I USE ON HEMORRHOIDS BEFORE SENDING A PATIENT TO THE SURGEON?

Brian E. Lacy, MD, PhD

Although common, hemorrhoids are widely misunderstood by both patients and physicians. They are mistakenly blamed for a variety of perianal symptoms and are frequently confused with other perianal disorders. A thorough understanding of the pathophysiology of hemorrhoids is essential if appropriate treatment is to be provided. Hemorrhoids have a prevalence rate of approximately 4%, affect men and women equally, and increase in incidence with age.[1] The natural history of hemorrhoids has not been well studied.

A cushion of tissue lies beneath the mucosa of the anal canal. This cushion, supported by smooth muscle, consists of connective tissue and an extensive arteriovenous plexus. This vascular plexus is supplied by the superior rectal artery and drained by the inferior, middle, and superior rectal veins. Congestion and dilation of the arteriovenous plexus leads to the development of hemorrhoids. The dentate line is an important landmark, because internal hemorrhoids reside above the dentate line, while external hemorrhoids lie below. The dentate line is also an important marker for pain, as the area above the dentate line is poorly innervated, while the area below the dentate line is exquisitely innervated, and irritation of this area may be associated with significant pain. Hemorrhoids are classified based on bleeding and prolapse. First-degree hemorrhoids bleed but do not prolapse, while second-degree hemorrhoids prolapse but reduce spontaneously. Third-degree hemorrhoids prolapse and require manual assistance to reduce them, while fourth-degree hemorrhoids cannot be reduced and thus are prone to thrombosis and infarction.

The underlying cause of hemorrhoidal swelling and prolapse is not known. It is commonly believed that straining, chronic constipation, chronic diarrhea, and increased abdominal pressure (ie, pregnancy) all increase the likelihood of hemorrhoids developing, although no prospective studies have confirmed these views. Several studies have shown that anal canal pressures, measured by anorectal manometry, are higher in patients with hemorrhoids. These elevated pressures return to normal after hemorrhoidectomy. Prolapse likely occurs due to weakening of the connective tissue and smooth muscle support system that normally holds the arteriovenous plexus in place, although again, the precise cause is not known.

Contrary to popular opinion, external hemorrhoids do not itch or burn. On occasion, they may rupture, leading to bright red rectal bleeding. External hemorrhoids may thrombose, and patients typically complain of the sudden onset of anal pain with a sensation of a "lump" in the perianal region. Skin tags may develop after external hemorrhoidal rupture or thrombosis, and these can cause perianal hygiene problems in some patients with the subsequent development of pruritus ani.

As noted above, internal hemorrhoids may bleed or prolapse. Prolapse may lead to excess mucus and difficulties with hygiene, a prelude to pruritus ani in some patients. Bleeding is typically acute, bright red, and not associated with abdominal or anal pain.

A careful history and a good physical examination are paramount in the evaluation of patients with presumed hemorrhoidal symptoms.[1,2] The pain of a thrombosed external hemorrhoid can be confused with a fissure, although a careful physical examination can easily distinguish those possibilities. A fissure, however, can occur in up to 20% of patients with hemorrhoidal bleeding. Perianal growths, including condylomata acuminata and cancer, appear very different than the dilated, painful thrombosed hemorrhoid or the purplish mucosa of rectal prolapse. Evidence of excoriation and lichenification, consistent with pruritus ani, should be sought. Digital rectal examination will permit anal sphincter resting tone and squeeze pressure to be quickly measured as well as exclusion of rectal masses with a 360-degree sweep of the rectum with the examining finger. A complete blood count should be performed if not recently done, and an abdominal examination should be performed as well. Nearly all surgical and gastroenterology societies recommend anoscopy and flexible sigmoidoscopy in the evaluation of a patient with bright red rectal bleeding. Rectal varices, which are treated differently than internal hemorrhoids, can be identified at this time. Hemoccult cards do not have any value in patients with rectal bleeding and should not be used. In a younger patient (<40 years) without any warning signs (anemia, unintentional weight loss, family history of colorectal cancer or IBD, abnormal abdominal examination), no further evaluation is usually required. However, if symptoms persist despite treatment, if the clinical situation changes, or if warning signs are present, then colonoscopy is warranted.

Third- and fourth-degree hemorrhoids require surgery, and little time should be spent attempting to manage these patients more conservatively. Grade I and II hemorrhoids frequently improve with time and conservative therapy.[1,3] I use a step-wise approach when treating patients with hemorrhoids, based on clinical experience, as there are few prospective, well-designed, placebo-controlled studies to guide therapy. Patients are counseled to take in an adequate amount of fiber (25 to 30 g/day), because a recent meta-analysis demonstrated that supplemental fiber does reduce bleeding when compared to placebo.[3] Patients are asked to schedule routine bathroom time each day, typically 30 minutes after a meal, to take advantage of the natural gastrocolic reflex and to minimize straining. If present, constipation should be treated with any of the four Food and Drug Administration-approved medications. Diarrhea can be treated with loperamide or diphenoxylate. Sitz baths may help to relax the anal sphincter, thus promoting drainage of dilated vessels, while also helping to keep the perianal area clean. Topical nitrates reduce resting pressure of the anal canal but are unlikely to help with first- or second-degree hemorrhoids. Several studies have, however, shown that they improve healing after hemorrhoid surgery. Topical steroids may transiently improve symptoms, but they do not reduce hemorrhoids and chronic use can lead to thinning of the skin. Topical anesthetics (ie, lidocaine) can improve pain from a thrombosed hemorrhoid or treat symptoms of pruritus, but do not reduce hemorrhoidal swelling. Topical calcium channel blockers may reduce anal canal pressures, but again do not relieve hemorrhoidal swelling or bleeding. External hemorrhoids can generally be safely sclerosed with a variety of substances (salt water, phenol in oil), although ulceration and infection can occur. Internal hemorrhoids can be banded, and this should occur at least 2 cm above the dentate line in order to minimize pain. Cauterization of internal hemorrhoids, using either bipolar electrocoagulation or argon plasma coagulation, is effective in some patients. Cryotherapy has been largely abandoned due to complications. Although a variety of alternative medicines have been used, none have been carefully studied. Flavonoids are popular in Europe and Asia, and several studies have shown that these seem to reduce bleeding. They are generally sold in a micronized form for oral ingestion, MPFF (micronized purified flavonoid fraction).

References

1. Madoff RD, Fleshman JW, Clinical Practice Committee, American Gastroenterological Association. American Gastroenterological Association technical review on the diagnosis and treatment of hemorrhoids. *Gastroenterology*. 2004;126(5):1463-1473.
2. Tang T, Lim PB, Miller R. An approach to hemorrhoids. *Colorectal Dis*. 2005;7(2):143-147.
3. Alonso-Coello P, Mills E, Heels-Ansdell D, et al. Fiber for the treatment of hemorrhoids complications: a systematic review and meta-analysis. *Am J Gastroenterol*. 2006;101(1):181-188.

What Tips Can I Give My Surgical Colleagues Who Are Seeing Patients With Pouchitis?

L. Campbell Levy, MD
Corey A. Siegel, MD

Background and Risk Factors

Restorative proctocolectomy with ileal pouch-anal anastamosis (IPAA) is the surgical treatment of choice for patients with medically refractory ulcerative colitis (UC), for a complication of UC such as dysplasia or cancer, and for most patients with familial adenomatous polyposis syndrome.[1] Approximately 25% to 30% of patients with UC eventually require proctocolectomy. Possible complications after IPAA include Crohn's disease of the pouch, cuffitis, irritable pouch syndrome, and an idiopathic chronic inflammatory condition of the pouch referred to as pouchitis.[2] Pouchitis is the most common complication after IPAA for UC, occurring in up to 60% of patients. Forty percent of patients respond to treatment and never have another episode. Five percent to 20% of patients will have an intermittent or chronic course requiring protracted therapy.[2]

The etiology is not well known; genetic susceptibility, bacterial overgrowth, and/or imbalance of bacterial flora appear to be important factors.[3] Although there is some inconsistency between studies, risk factors for pouchitis include extensive UC, backwash ileitis, young age at diagnosis of UC, the presence of perinuclear antineutrophil cytoplasmic antibodies, nonsteroidal anti-inflammatory drug (NSAID) use, the presence of extraintestinal manifestations of inflammatory bowel disease, and primary sclerosing cholangitis.[1] The surgical technique used to construct the pouch does not affect the risk of pouchitis.[4]

Clinical Features and Diagnosis

The most common symptoms of pouchitis are increased stool frequency and liquidity, urgency, abdominal cramping, pelvic discomfort, and, more rarely in severe pouchitis, fever and/or rectal bleeding.[2] Given the high frequency of pouchitis after IPAA, some clinicians treat empirically based on symptoms. The most cost-effective approach is pouchoscopy without biopsies.[5] However, we prefer endoscopy with biopsies at initial presentation because it narrows the differential diagnosis, and it may distinguish pouchitis from Crohn's disease, CMV infection, ischemia, pyloric gland metaplasia, and functional disorders.[1] Endoscopic findings are consistent with inflammation and can be patchy or diffuse. The neoterminal ileum proximal to the pouch is not involved.[4] Ulcers around the staple line are common even in the absence of pouchitis, so we avoid taking biopsies in this area.[1] Symptoms do not necessarily correlate with the severity of endoscopic findings. Therefore, even if the pouch appears normal, we will take random biopsies to evaluate for active inflammation.[2] Lastly, we prefer using a gastroscope for pouchoscopy due to its increased flexibility and maneuverability.

Medical Therapies

Despite a relative lack of randomized controlled trials, antibiotics remain the mainstay of therapy for pouchitis. In our experience, most patients respond to therapy within the first 2 days of a treatment course, which consists of 10 to 14 days of metronidazole 750 to 1000 mg/day or ciprofloxacin 1000 mg/day.[1] A trial comparing ciprofloxacin to metronidazole showed significant improvements in symptom, histologic, and endoscopic scores with both drugs. However, because patients taking ciprofloxacin had fewer adverse effects and a greater reduction in symptom scores, ciprofloxacin is most often our initial treatment of choice.[6] If patients are initially started on metronidazole and do not respond, they may respond to ciprofloxacin and/or combination therapy. There are uncontrolled data for other antibiotics including rifaximin, erythromycin, topical metronidazole, amoxicillin/clavulanate, and tetracycline. Our early experience with rifaximin has so far been promising.[1]

Some patients may develop chronic or relapsing pouchitis that may require low-dose maintenance or pulse antibiotic therapy. In patients who are unresponsive to standard antibiotics, alternative treatment options without much supportive data include topical or oral 5-aminosalicilates, topical or oral steroids (including budesonide), bismuth, and allopurinol. For refractory cases we also consider immunomodulators, such as azathioprine or 6-mercaptopurine. There are case reports that suggest a possible utility of infliximab.

Probiotics have been found to be safe and effective for the treatment and prevention of pouchitis. In a randomized controlled trial of patients with recurrent or refractory pouchitis, VSL #3 maintained remission more often than placebo (85% in VLS #3 group vs 6% placebo).[7] Therefore, we recommend VSL #3 to this group of patients. When given at the time of ileostomy take-down after IPAA, VSL #3 appears to prevent the onset of pouchitis (10% VSL #3 group vs 40% placebo).[8] Although further studies are warranted, the use of probiotics appears to be safe and effective for the treatment and prevention of pouchitis.

When Medical Therapy Fails

A small minority of patients with pouchitis fail medical therapy. In one study of 100 consecutive patients who underwent IPAA, only 2 required pouch resection.[2] Prior to referral for surgery, we systematically evaluate for other possible etiologies for the patient's symptoms. Though *Clostridium difficile* is a rare cause of inflammation of the pouch, we will measure a stool antigen. Pouchoscopy with biopsies should also be conducted to evaluate for CMV pouchitis and Crohn's disease. Approximately 5% of patients with a diagnosis of UC prior to IPAA have Crohn's disease based on review of pre- and postoperative pathology specimens.[2] After excluding alternative diagnoses in patients with pouchitis refractory to standard therapy, the risk and benefits of further medical options should be weighed against proceeding with permanent ileostomy with excision or exclusion of the pouch. We attempt to individualize these risks to patients in concert with consultation from our most experienced colorectal surgery colleagues. If further medical treatments fail or if patients prefer not to continue with medical therapy, then they should be referred for surgery.

References

1. Pardi DS, Sandborn WJ. Systematic review: the management of pouchitis. *Aliment Pharmacol Ther.* 2006;23(8):1087-1096.
2. Shen B, Fazio VW, Remzi FH, Lashner BA. Clinical approach to disease of ileal pouch-anal anastomosis. *Am J Gastroenterol.* 2005;100(12):2796-2807.
3. Lim M, Sagar P, Finan P, Burke D, Schuster H. Dysbiosis and pouchitis. *Br J Surg.* 2006;93(11):1325-1334.
4. Gionchetti P, Morselli C, Rizzello F, et al. Management of pouch dysfunction or pouchitis with an ileoanal pouch. *Best Pract Res Clin Gastroenterol.* 2004;18(5):993-1006.
5. Shen B, Shermock KM, Fazio VW, et al. A cost-effectiveness analysis of diagnostic strategies for symptomatic patients with ileal pouch-anal anastomosis. *Am J Gastroenterol.* 2003;98(11):2460-2467.
6. Shen B, Achkar JP, Lashner BA, et al. A randomized clinical trial of ciprofloxacin and metronidazole to treat acute pouchitis. *Inflamm Bowel Dis.* 2001;7(4):301-305.
7. Mimura T, Rizzello F, Helwig U, et al. Once daily high dose probiotic therapy (VSL #3) for maintaining remission in recurrent or refractory pouchitis. *Gut.* 2004;53(1):108-114.
8. Gionchetti P, Rizzello F, Helwig U, et al. Prophylaxis of pouchitis onset with probiotic therapy: a double-blind placebo controlled trial. *Gastroenterology.* 2003;124(5):1202-1209.

A 74-Year-Old Man Who Is Status Post External Radiation Therapy for Prostate Cancer Now Presents With Hematochezia. What Should I Do Next? Can I Keep This From Recurring?

Brian E. Lacy, MD, PhD

Prostate cancer is commonly treated with radiation therapy, which can be associated with significant morbidity. The degree and extent of radiation injury depends upon the dose of radiation provided, the location of the radiation (internal vs external), the use of shielding, changes in radiation orientation, the extent of bladder filling, the interval between sessions, and the overall health and nutritional status of the patient at the time of radiation. Combination external beam therapy and implant therapy is more likely to produce injury than either type of therapy alone. Although the colon is considered relatively resistant to radiation-induced injury, the rectum and sigmoid colon are at increased risk due to their location and relative immobility. External beam radiation therapy, as opposed to implant therapy, is more likely to produce complications, which include superficial burns, the development of a rectovaginal or colocutaneous fistula, urethral strictures, rectal stenosis, and cystitis. More importantly, up to 30% of patients who undergo radiation therapy for prostate cancer will develop radiation proctitis.[1] This can occur in one of two forms, acute or chronic.

Acute radiation proctitis develops either during therapy or within 4 to 6 weeks of completing therapy. Patients may complain of excessive mucus with stools, feelings of urgency and tenesmus, lower abdominal pain, and occasionally rectal bleeding. Endoscopic evaluation may be completely normal or may reveal fairly nonspecific findings of pale mucosa with areas of erythema. Biopsies are generally nonspecific, and symptoms generally resolve spontaneously. Approximately 20% of patients with acute radiation proctitis will develop chronic symptoms.

Chronic radiation proctitis may develop from 1 to 30 years after completion of radiation therapy, although most patients first note symptoms 1 to 2 years after therapy. Hematochezia is common; patients may also have symptoms of urgency, tenesmus, excessive passage of mucus, and rectal pain. Only a small percentage of patients require transfusions, although those who do are more likely to have a prolonged course, have other complications, and have an increased mortality rate. Endoscopic changes are characteristic, revealing pale mucosa and telangiectasias; ulcers may occasionally be seen. Biopsies may reveal fibrosis of the connective tissue along with platelet thrombi in arterioles and subintimal fibrosis.

Patients with acute radiation proctitis can generally be managed conservatively without any diagnostic testing. Many patients note some improvement in symptoms of urgency and mucus by eliminating or reducing caffeine, dairy, fructose, and fiber from their diet. If symptoms persist, stool samples should be ordered to look for a coexisting infection. Severe symptoms warrant a delay in radiation therapy, which usually leads to an improvement in symptoms. Persistent symptoms and hematochezia necessitate diagnostic evaluation, as described below.

Patients with obstructive symptoms should undergo flexible sigmoidoscopy combined with a barium enema or a full colonoscopy. Short strictures that are mild can be dilated using a transendoscopic balloon. Biopsies should be taken to rule out malignancy. Long, tight strictures will not respond to sequential dilation and will require surgery. Primary anastomosis can be performed at the time of surgical resection. At least one side of the anastomosis should be free of radiation injury to minimize the chance of an anastomotic leak.

Flexible sigmoidoscopy should be the first test performed in those patients with hematochezia. If bleeding continues, and sigmoidoscopy is normal, then colonoscopy should be performed. If characteristic changes of radiation-induced injury are seen (pallor and telangiectasias), biopsies are not required. If bleeding continues despite a normal colonoscopy, then a video capsule study should be performed to look for radiation-induced injury to the small intestine. Brisk bleeding should be evaluated with a tagged red blood cell scan. In the absence of upper gastrointestinal symptoms, upper endoscopy has little value.

Patients with mild intermittent hematochezia without anemia or the need for transfusion can be safely treated with topical medications. However, the efficacy of most topical medications, including sulfasalazine and 5-ASA preparations, is limited. Topical steroids may improve mild symptoms in some patients, but most studies are not encouraging. Sucralfate enemas (2 to 3 g daily for 2 to 4 weeks) have been shown to reduce bleeding and symptoms of tenesmus and mucus in several small studies. Combining topical sucralfate with oral sucralfate (1 g orally 4 times daily) may further improve symptoms. Short-chain fatty acids have not been shown to improve symptoms of radiation proctitis. Topical formalin has been used to improve symptoms in radiation-induced cystitis.[2] A number of studies, involving small numbers of patients, demonstrated that formalin instillation improved hematochezia and reduced the need for blood transfusions. However, instillation can be difficult and, if improperly applied, may cause severe perianal dermatitis. Other researchers have used formalin-soaked gauze (4% solution) applied topically to each of the 4 quadrants in the rectum. Patients generally require 2 to 4 treatment sessions, and most note a significant reduction in bleeding.

Persistent symptoms that fail to respond to conservative topical therapy require endoscopic therapy. Laser therapy (Nd:YAG—neodymium yttrium-aluminum-garnet) was first used in the early 1980s. Several studies have shown that it is safe and effective. The tip is applied close to, but not touching, the mucosa. Most clinicians use 40 W with 0.5 second pulse durations. Visible lesions should be coagulated, working from the proximal to distal direction. Most patients will require several treatment sessions. Argon plasma coagulation (APC) has replaced Nd:YAG in most centers, because it is cheaper, safer, and easier to use.[3] High-frequency energy applied to the rectal mucosa through the ionized argon coagulates the hemorrhagic areas. Settings range from 50 to 60 W at a flow rate of 1.5 to 3 L/min. Most patients will require several sessions. A number of studies have shown that APC significantly reduces the number of bleeding episodes.

Although only available at a few academic centers, hyperbaric oxygen therapy has shown promising results in small studies.[4] Larger studies are required to confirm these initial encouraging results.

References

1. Ajlouni M. Radiation-induced proctitis. *Curr Treat Options Gastroenterol.* 1999;2(1):20-26.
2. Tsujinaka S, Baig MK, Gornev R, et al. Formalin instillation for hemorrhagic radiation proctitis. *Surg Innov.* 2005;12(2):123-128.
3. Fantin AC, Binek J, Suter WR, Meyenberger C. Argon beam coagulation for treatment of symptomatic radiation-induced proctitis. *Gastrointest Endosc.* 1999;49(4 Pt 1):515-518.
4. Woo TC, Joseph D, Oxer H. Hyperbaric oxygen treatment for radiation proctitis. *Int J Radiat Oncol Biol Phys.* 1997;38(3):619-622.

WHAT SHOULD BE THE SEQUENCE OF INVESTIGATIONS FOR A PATIENT WITH RECTAL ADENOCARCINOMA?

Brian E. Lacy, MD, PhD

Of the nearly 150,000 Americans diagnosed with colorectal cancer per year, approximately 42,000 will have rectal adenocarcinoma. Most patients with rectal cancer are asymptomatic and the disease is diagnosed via colorectal cancer screening.[1] Rectal cancer can spread by direct invasion, through lymphatics, or via hematogenous dissemination. The most common sites for metastases to occur are the liver, lungs, peritoneum, and bone. Accurate staging determines the therapeutic approach to rectal cancer, and the following steps should be followed to optimize staging.

Pathology specimens obtained during either flexible sigmoidoscopy or colonoscopy should be reviewed by two separate pathologists to confirm the diagnosis.[2] A careful digital rectal examination should be performed in all patients to determine the distal extent of the lesion, possible involvement of the anal sphincters, and whether the tumor is fixed to the pelvic wall. Abdominal examination should be performed, as should an abdominal x-ray if symptoms of obstruction are present. "Clearance" of the colon of synchronous lesions proximal to the tumor with colonoscopy in patients diagnosed via sigmoidoscopy should be performed. If an obstructing lesion prohibits examination of the colon proximal to the lesion, then computer tomographic colonography or barium enema should be performed.[2] Patients with a history of hematochezia, unintentional weight loss, or weakness should have a complete blood count (CBC) checked.

The staging system that is most widely recognized is the TNM (Tumor, Node, Metastases) system of the American Joint Committee on Cancer. The numbers in parentheses after each description signify the distribution of disease in the United States and the 5-year survival rate.[3] TNM-I signifies that the tumor is localized to the mucosa and/or submucosa (34%; 80% to 90%). TNM-II indicates that the tumor extends into or through the muscle layer (25%; 50% to 60%). TNM-III means that lymph node involvement has occurred (26%); this was recently subdivided into A, B, and C categories, with 5-year survival rates ranging from 55% for TNM-IIIA to 24.5% for TNM-IIIC. TNM-IV means that distant metastases are present (15%; <5%).

A chest x-ray should be performed in all patients to look for pulmonary metastases.[4] Endoscopic endorectal ultrasound is better than magnetic resonance imaging at evaluating the depth of tumor invasion and should be performed. Many authorities believe that if the tumor is a TNM-I lesion, a CT scan of the pelvis and abdomen is not required; however, most practitioners routinely order a CT scan of the abdomen and pelvis with oral and intravenous contrast in all patients with rectal adenocarcinoma. Of note, pelvic CT scans are accurate in detecting lymph node involvement in only 60% of the cases.[5] A carcinoembryonic antigen (CEA) level should be checked in all patients who will require surgery, and CEA levels >5 ng/mL impart a worse prognosis. Finally, prior to surgery, nearly all surgeons perform rigid sigmoidoscopy to determine the distance of the most distant part of the lesion from the dentate line. This landmark is considered more reliable and accurate than the anal verge.

References

1. Speights VO, Johnson MW, Stoltenberg PH, Rappaport ES, Helbert B, Riggs M. Colorectal cancer: current trends in initial clinical manifestations. *South Med J.* 1991;84(5):575-578.
2. Jessup JM, Stewart AK, Menck HR. The National Cancer Data Base report on patterns of care for adenocarcinoma of the rectum, 1985-1995. *Cancer.* 1998;83(11):2408-2418.
3. Minsky BD, Mies C, Recht A, Rich TA, Chaffey JT. Resectable adenocarcinoma of the rectosigmoid and rectum. Patterns of failure and survival. *Cancer.* 1988;61(7):1408.
4. Sauer R, Becker H, Hohenberger W, et al. Preoperative versus postoperative chemoradiotherapy for rectal cancer. *N Engl J Med.* 2004;351(17):1731-1740.
5. Chen ET, Mohiuddin M, Brodovsky H, Fishbein G, Marks G. Downstaging of advanced rectal cancer following combined preoperative chemotherapy and high dose radiation. *Int J Radiat Oncol Biol Phys.* 1994;30(1):169.

WHAT IS SOLITARY RECTAL ULCER SYNDROME?

Brian E. Lacy, MD, PhD

Solitary rectal ulcer syndrome (SRUS) was first recognized as a distinct clinical entity in 1969 with the description of 68 cases.[1] It is a benign disorder of young adults, although it has been identified in young children and in the elderly. It is an uncommon disorder with an incidence of approximately 1 in 100,000 people per year.[2] The average age of diagnosis is in the third to fourth decade of life. Women are somewhat more prone to develop SRUS than men; race and socioeconomic status do not seem to play a role.

SRUS is actually a misnomer, because only 25% to 30% of patients have a single ulcer. Thirty percent of patients have multiple ulcers, while others have hyperemic mucosa or polypoid lesions. Ulcers generally occur 4 to 10 cm from the anal verge, are more common on the anterior wall, and range in size from 0.5 to 6 cm, although most are 1 to 1.5 cm in diameter. Endoscopically, SRUS may appear as a hyperemic area, a punched-out isolated ulcer, or an ulcer with a hyperemic base and mucus. Some ulcers have rolled edges, or are polypoid in nature and, when bleeding, raise concern over a possible malignancy.

Symptoms of SRUS are nonspecific, which frequently leads to misdiagnosis or a delay in diagnosis.[3] Rectal bleeding and the passage of mucus are the two most commonly reported symptoms. Bleeding is typically just a small amount of blood with bowel movements, although it can be severe and require transfusions. Other frequently reported symptoms include straining at stool, feelings of incomplete evacuation, rectal discomfort, and urgency.

The precise cause of SRUS is not known, and several theories appear reasonable.[3] These theories include pressure necrosis, ischemia, and local trauma. Straining at stool can produce prolapse of rectal mucosa. During straining, increased abdominal pressure may cause the anterior rectal wall to press against the opposing wall. Recurrent pressure may produce an ulcer, or the persistent pressure may cause localized ischemia, with subsequent development of an ulcer. Persistent straining, especially in patients with pelvic floor dyssynergia, may reduce blood flow and directly lead to ischemia. Alternatively, some authorities believe that SRUS develops due to repeated trauma to the anorectal area, which may occur during digital stimulation or disimpaction. However, this theory has been discounted by other researchers, as the location of the ulcer is usually beyond the reach of an examining finger and because rates of SRUS are not higher in patients who require digital stimulation in order to effectively evacuate stool. Medications and infections have also been impugned; however, there are little data to support these latter theories.

Although a careful and thoughtful history is important for any patient with rectal bleeding, the different diagnosis is fairly broad at the outset. Younger adults with complaints of straining at stool and the passage of mucus, in addition to rectal bleeding, need to be considered for SRUS. The absence of severe rectal pain makes an anal fissure unlikely. If extra-intestinal manifestations of inflammatory bowel disease (iritis, uveitis, joint effusions, rash, family history of IBD, chronic diarrhea, bloody stools, anemia, and weight loss) are not present and a fissure is not present on examination, Crohn's disease is unlikely. Colorectal cancer is of great concern to patients, but the absence of a family history of colorectal cancer, and the absence of unintentional weight loss and anemia should be reassuring to the patient. Proctalgia fugax is characterized by fleeting rectal pain without bleeding, while levator ani syndrome is typified by rectal discomfort or a "lump" or "ball-like" sensation in the rectum without bleeding. A careful examination of the perianal region and rectum can exclude common anorectal disorders associated with bleeding, which include hemorrhoids, fissures, or a localized mass. Infections (syphilis, lymphogranuloma venereum, amebiasis), chronic ischemia, trauma, colitis cystica profunda, and a stercoral ulcer should also be considered.

In the absence of warning signs, flexible sigmoidoscopy should be performed to identify the characteristic lesion (see above). Biopsies need to be taken to exclude malignancy. Characteristic histologic features of SRUS include smooth muscle hyperplasia of the lamina propria with infiltration of collagen (aka "fibromuscular obliteration"), distortion of the crypt architecture, disorientation and thickening of the muscularis mucosa, and an increase in mucus cells with gland dilation. In patients with a history of significant straining, anorectal manometry and balloon expulsion should be performed to identify patients with pelvic floor dyssynergia. If present, the patients should be enrolled in a pelvic floor retraining program. Defecography (either with barium or using MRI) can be useful to identify prolapse and/or intussusception, but is not mandatory. Barium enemas are not clinically useful in the evaluation of SRUS. Transrectal ultrasound should be reserved for those patients who fail therapy and malignancy remains in the differential diagnosis.

The first treatment step is to educate the patient about the condition and to have the patient incorporate behaviors that can promote healing and decrease the likelihood of SRUS recurring. I ask patients to incorporate scheduled bathroom time into their daily routine with the goal of eliminating straining. This is best scheduled approximately 30 minutes after a meal, to take advantage of the natural gastrocolic reflex. Patients are taught Kegel exercises and proper evacuation techniques. A prospective study has shown that biofeedback improves healing.[4] The patient's diet should be reviewed to ensure that an adequate amount of fiber (25 to 30 g per day) is present. If not, supplemental fiber should be provided. Enemas (steroids, sulfasalazine, 5-aminosalicylate) are employed by many clinicians, although there are no data to support their use. Carafate enemas improved healing in one small, open label study. I avoid using stimulant laxatives, although patients with persistent symptoms of constipation, who may also have coexisting mild colonic inertia, may require treatment with polyethylene glycol or lubiprostone. Some clinicians inject the ulcer with steroids to improve healing, although no prospective controlled trials are available to determine if this is effective. Surgery is rarely required and should be reserved for those with persistent bleeding requiring transfusions or when biopsies raise the definite possibility of a malignancy.

References

1. Madigan MR, Morson BC. Solitary ulcer of the rectum. *Gut.* 1969;10(11):871-881.
2. Martin CJ, Parks TG, Biggart JD. Solitary rectal ulcer syndrome in Northern Ireland. 1971-1980. *Br J Surg.* 1981;68(10):744-747.
3. Tjandra JJ, Fazio VW, Church JM, Lavery IC, Oakley JR, Milsom JW. Clinical conundrum of solitary rectal ulcer. *Dis Colon Rectum.* 1992;35(3):227-234.
4. Rao SS, Ozturk R, De Ocampo S, Stessman M. Pathophysiology and role of biofeedback therapy in solitary rectal ulcer syndrome. *Am J Gastroenterol.* 2006;101(3):613-618.

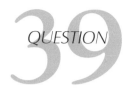

WHAT IS RECTAL PROLAPSE?

Brian E. Lacy, MD, PhD

Primary causes of constipation include obstructed defecation, irritable bowel syndrome, colonic inertia, and normal transit constipation. Of the large group of disorders that cause obstructed defecation, rectal prolapse is one of the two most common reasons (the other being internal mucosal prolapse). Rectal prolapse (procidentia) is defined as a protrusion of the rectum beyond the anus.[1] Full-thickness or complete rectal prolapse is the protrusion of all of the layers of the rectal wall beyond the anus. Mucosal prolapse (incomplete prolapse) is the protrusion of only the rectal mucosa. Internal prolapse or rectal intussusception is prolapse of the rectal wall that does not extend beyond the anus.

Rectal prolapse is primarily a disorder of older adults. Women are much more likely to be affected than men, and the incidence rises through the fifth and sixth decades of life until it peaks in the seventh decade. Children can also be affected, likely due to a congenital defect, although those with cystic fibrosis, whooping cough, and tuberculosis are also at increased risk. Risk factors for developing rectal prolapse in adults include constipation, prior childbirth, multiple and prolonged childbirths, obstetric trauma, prostate enlargement, scleroderma, and other connective tissue disorders.

Initial symptoms of rectal prolapse include straining at stool and a sense of partial obstruction, which may be intermittent at first. Patients frequently have feelings of incomplete evacuation and tenesmus, in addition to symptoms of excessive mucus per rectum. As the prolapse worsens, bleeding may occur. Patients may sense a "mass" in the rectal area, which is worrisome for cancer. Longstanding prolapse may lead to fecal incontinence.

A number of theories have been proposed to explain the development of rectal prolapse.[2] Unfortunately, despite a number of well-designed studies, significant controversy remains. Nearly all authorities agree, however, that a lax pelvic floor is a prerequisite to the development of prolapse. A mobile mesorectum, weak lateral ligaments, and weak sphincter muscles (both internal and external) also likely contribute to the development of prolapse. Pudendal nerve neuropathy, due to compression or stretching during childbirth, and an abnormally large pouch of Douglas, may also play a role.

A careful physical examination of the anorectal area is the first step in the evaluation of patients with possible rectal prolapse. Inspection of the anorectal area can quickly differentiate other disorders that cause bleeding (fissures, hemorrhoids, a rectal mass) or also produce symptoms of fullness and incomplete evacuation (rectocele, descending perineum syndrome). If not already evident, full-thickness or mucosal prolapse can be demonstrated by having the patient perform a Valsalva maneuver during examination of the anorectal area. Internal prolapse can be felt during examination of the rectal canal as a fold of tissue strikes the examining finger with straining. Because prolapse is most common in the older population where colon cancer rates are highest, colonoscopy should be performed to rule out other sources of bleeding (colorectal cancer, arteriovenous malformations, solitary rectal ulcer syndrome, internal hemorrhoids, and diverticulosis). If prolapse is not evident or cannot be produced during the examination, then defecography (either video or MRI) can be employed. Patients who require surgery should have preoperative anorectal manometry performed, which typically reveals low sphincter pressures.

The goals of treatment are fourfold: reduce the prolapse, prevent prolapse from recurring, restore or maintain continence, and prevent straining and constipation. Medical therapy is useful in some patients with mild dysfunction and internal prolapse. Adding more fiber to the diet and enrolling the patient in a biofeedback program to minimize straining and improve evacuation may resolve or minimize symptoms in a small percentage of patients. However, most patients with prolapse will eventually require surgery.

The therapeutic goals noted above can be achieved surgically by resecting the redundant rectum, plicating the redundant folds of tissue, or permanently attaching the rectum to the sacrum to prevent excessive movement. Surgery can be performed using an abdominal approach (either open or laparoscopic) or a perineal approach. The former approach is preferred in younger, healthier patients, while the latter is preferred in older, less healthy patients. Rectopexy involves mobilizing the rectum and relocating it to a more superior position.[3] Scar tissue, produced by the placement of sutures or mesh, eventually leads to fixation of the rectum to the sacrum. Alternatively, an anterior sling rectopexy can be performed (Ripstein procedure) during which synthetic material is placed in front of the rectum and sutured to the sacral promontory. This fixes the rectum in place and restores its normal anatomic position. Resection of the rectosigmoid colon (resection-rectopexy; Frykman-Goldberg procedure) is an alternative for some patients because it removes redundant tissue, straightens the left colon, improves constipation (in some patients), and fixes the rectum onto the sacrum as scar tissue forms. The Delorme procedure is one of the most common perineal procedures performed. During this operation, the rectal mucosa is stripped, the muscular layer is plicated to reduce redundant tissue, and the mucosa is reattached to cover the plicated tissue. Perineal rectosigmoidectomy can also be performed, and may be better suited for the more fragile patient than an abdominal approach. No studies have compared these surgical techniques in a prospective manner.

References

1 Wassef R, Rothenberger DA, Goldberg SM. Rectal prolapse. *Curr Probl Surg.* 1986;23(6):397-451.
2. Sun WM, Read NW, Donnelly TC, Bannister JJ, Shorthouse AJ. A common pathophysiology for full thickness rectal prolapse, anterior mucosal prolapse, and solitary rectal ulcer. *Br J Surg.* 1989;76(3):290-295.
3. Poen AC, de Brauw M, Felt-Bersma RJ, de Jong D, Cuesta MA. Laparoscopic rectopexy for complete rectal prolapse. Clinical outcome and anorectal function tests. *Surg Endosc.* 1996;10(9):904-908.

SECTION V

COLON POTPOURRI

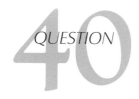

THE EMERGENCY ROOM IS CALLING ABOUT A PATIENT WITH PNEUMATOSIS COLI. WHAT DO I NEED TO DO?

Inku Hwang, MD

Pneumatosis coli (also known by such names as pneumatosis intestinalis, pneumatosis cystoides intestinalis, and intestinal emphysema) is a condition that involves the presence of gas within the wall of the colon (Figure 40-1). The more generic term pneumatosis intestinalis implies air in either the small or large bowel. This in itself is not a diagnosis but a sign of other diseases. The exact incidence is unknown because it is often found incidentally in asymptomatic patients, but it can be found in patients of all ages.[1] In children, it is most often associated with necrotizing enterocolitis. In adults, it is more often seen in the elderly and may be due to various medical conditions including severe intra-abdominal diseases, infections, chronic gastrointestinal diseases, pulmonary diseases, and various other conditions affecting gastrointestinal motility and the immune system (Table 40-1).[2,3]

The most important issue for the emergency room is to determine whether the patient is symptomatic, and whether the symptoms suggest an underlying surgical abdomen. If so, this patient should undergo an emergent surgery consultation. If not, the patient should be further evaluated for possible underlying causes of the pneumatosis coli and be treated appropriately.

Patients with pneumatosis may have no symptoms, have symptoms of the underlying diseases listed above, or have symptoms from pneumatosis itself. If the symptoms are due to the pneumatosis, the presenting symptom is usually dependent on where the air is located. For pneumatosis in the small bowel, patients present most commonly with vomiting, followed in order of frequency by abdominal distension, weight loss, abdominal pain, and diarrhea.[4] With colonic pneumatosis, the most common symptom is diarrhea, followed in order of frequency by hematochezia, abdominal pain, abdominal distension, and constipation. Physical exam is often not helpful in diagnosing these patients. Computed tomography (CT) may be the most helpful as it is more sensitive

Figure 40-1. Pneumatosis coli evident on (A) abdominal plain film and (B) abdominal CT scan depicting the presence of intramural gas in the colon.

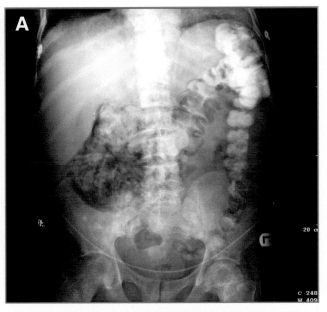

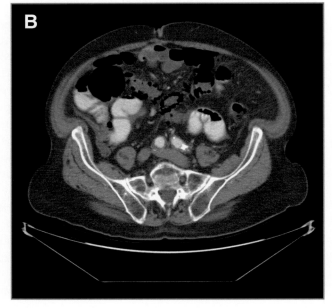

than plain film abdominal imaging, and it may give additional information about underlying causes.

The medical management of patients with nonsurgical pneumatosis includes oxygen therapy (inhaled or hyperbaric), antibiotics, and even endoscopy. However, for approximately 15% of adult patients with pneumatosis coli, no obvious etiology of the condition will be identified. The majority of these patients will have a benign course and will require no therapy.[2]

Table 40-1
Causes of Pneumatosis Intestinalis[5]

Surgical Emergencies	*Diseases Affecting Gastrointestinal Motility*	*Infections*
• Intestinal ischemia • Intestinal infarction • Intestinal perforation • Intestinal obstruction • Necrotizing enterocolitis • Typhlitis	• Diabetes • Scleroderma • Hirschsprung's disease • Intestinal pseudo-obstruction • Jejunoileal bypass • Pyloric stenosis/obstruction	• *Clostridium difficile* • Tuberculosis • Whipple's disease • AIDS entrocolitides • Cryptosporidium • *Mycobacterium avium* • Intracellulare • CMV
Mucosal Disruption • Peptic ulcer disease • Crohn's disease • Ulcerative colitis • Feeding jejunostomy tube • Caustic ingestions • Ruptured diverticulum	*Immunological Disturbances* • AIDS • Steroids • Chemotherapy • Lymphoproliferative disorders • Bone marrow transplantation • Solid organ transplantation • Graft versus host disease • Amyloidosis • Collagen vascular disease	*Pulmonary Disorders* • Chronic obstructive pulmonary disease • Asthma • Cystic fibrosis • Mechanical ventilation
Endoscopic Procedures • EGD • Colonoscopy • Sclerotherapy • Biliary stent placement		

References

1. Heng Y, Schuffler MD, Haggitt RC, Rohrmann CA. Pneumatosis intestinalis: a review. *Am J Gastroenterol.* 1995;90(10):1747-1758.
2. Knechtle SJ, Davidoff AM, Rice RP. Pneumatosis intestinalis. Surgical management and clinical outcome. *Ann Surg.* 1990;212(2):160-165.
3. Koss LG. Abdominal gas cysts (pneumatosis cystoides intestinorum hominis); an analysis with a report of a case and a critical review of the literature. *AMA Arch Pathol.* 1952;53(6):523-549.
4. Jamart J. Pneumatosis cystoides intestinalis. A statistical study of 919 cases. *Acta Hepatogastroenterol (Stuttg).* 1979;26(5):419-422.
5. Goldberg E, LaMont JT. Pneumatosis intestinalis. *UpToDate.* 2005.

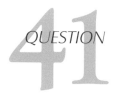

WHAT IS THE APPROPRIATE EVALUATION FOR FECAL INCONTINENCE?

Inku Hwang, MD

Fecal incontinence is a common problem affecting up to 15% of adults living in the general community[1] and nearly half of adults living in nursing homes.[2] However, the actual prevalence is likely underestimated given the social stigma associated with it, and for those affected, it can significantly impact their lives.

In order to understand fecal incontinence, we need to understand the physiology of fecal continence, which involves the coordinated function of several neuromuscular events.[3] In normal individuals, the colon receives approximately 800 mL of liquid stool from the terminal ileum, and this stool is moved by peristalsis to and fro in the colon until all but about 100 mL of the liquid has been reabsorbed and a solid stool residue has accumulated in preparation for evacuation. Several times a day a mass contraction wave moves through the colon, propelling the solid stool toward the rectum. As the rectum distends beyond approximately 300 mL, rectal pressure begins to increase and the urge to defecate occurs. The normally contracted internal anal sphincter reflexively relaxes and the rectum contracts, allowing the stool bolus to be eliminated. This last phase is subject to voluntary control after toilet training during childhood, and is coordinated with the relaxation of the external anal sphincter and the puborectalis sling. When necessary, the external anal sphincter and puborectalis sling can be consciously contracted to create pressures above the intrarectal pressure in order to prevent stool from being released accidently. In addition, the very distal rectum and proximal anus are richly populated with sensory neurons that permit the discrimination between liquid, solid, and gas so that individuals with normal bowel function are able to distinguish between flatus, liquid, and solid stool. It is when these mechanisms fail with inadequate external anal sphincter pressure, insufficient puborectalis function, inadequate rectal compliance, or inability to sense an impending bowel movement, that fecal incontinence can occur.

All patients with fecal incontinence should receive a careful history and physical exam. The history should focus on frequency, volume, and consistency of the stools and the severity of incontinence (ie, whether there is leakage of stools or full loss of bowel

Table 41-1

Tests for Fecal Incontinence

Test	*How Test Is Done*	*What Test Looks For*
Anorectal manometry	Small, pressure-sensitive catheter with a balloon at the tip is inserted into the rectum and withdrawn to measure the pressure of the anal sphincter. The balloon is inflated in incrementally larger volumes in the rectum to determine volume at which patient senses distension and to look for anorectal inhibitory reflex (ie, relaxation of the internal anal sphincter with rectal distension).	Resting tone of the internal anal sphincter Squeeze pressure of the external anal sphincter Threshold volume for conscious rectal sensation Anorectal inhibitory reflex
Balloon expulsion test	Balloon is inserted into the rectum and filled with 50 mL of water; the patient is asked to evacuate the balloon as if having a bowel movement.	Pelvic floor dyssynergia (lack of coordination between pelvic floor, anal sphincter, and abdominal muscles during bowel movement)
Endorectal ultrasound	Ultrasound probe is inserted into the anal canal, and the layers of the anal sphincter are examined for evidence of sphincter injury.	Anal sphincter injury that may be amenable to surgical repair
Endorectal MRI	Small MRI coil is placed in the anal canal, and the layers of the anal sphincter are examined for evidence of sphincter injury.	Anal sphincter injury that may be amenable to surgical repair
Pudendal nerve terminal latency	Pudendal nerve is stimulated, and time from stimulation to external anal sphincter contraction is measured.	Damage to the pudendal nerve
Electromyography	Electrode placed at anal sphincter is stimulated to determine muscular activity of the anal sphincter.	Muscular function of the anal sphincter
Defecography	Barium paste is instilled into the rectum, and the patient sits on a radiolucent commode to evacuate. Using fluoroscopy, anatomic changes during defecation are visualized.	Measures the anorectal angle and pelvic floor descent during defecation Anatomic defects in the anus and rectum detected

control). The medical history should be carefully reviewed to identify medical conditions that could be causing obstruction with overflow incontinence, mucosal inflammation, or neuromuscular conditions. The physical exam should involve a detailed anorectal exam, including a digital rectal exam.

Colonoscopy to exclude organic gastrointestinal disease is generally among the first diagnostic tests recommended for patients with fecal incontinence. Following that, there are various other tests available[4,5] (Table 41-1). However, subsequent tests should be carefully chosen with a specific therapy in mind because treatment options are limited to regulating stool texture or bowel habits, pelvic floor retraining, and surgery to repair the anal sphincter.[6]

References

1. Macmillan AK, Merrie AE, Marshall RJ, Parry BR. The prevalence of fecal incontinence in community-dwelling adults: a systematic review of the literature. *Dis Colon Rectum.* 2004;47(8):1341-1349.
2. Nelson R, Furner S, Jesudason V. Fecal incontinence in Wisconsin nursing homes: prevalence and associations. *Dis Colon Rectum.* 1998;41(10):1226-1229.
3. Sagar PM, Pemberton JH. Anorectal and pelvic floor function. Relevance of continence, incontinence, and constipation. *Gastroenterol Clin North Am.* 1996;25(1):163-182.
4. Bharucha AE, Wald A. Debate: anorectal manometry and imaging are necessary in patients with fecal incontinence. *Am J Gastroenterol.* 2006;101:2679-2684.
5. Diamant NE, Kamm MA, Wald A, Whitehead WE. AGA technical review on anorectal testing techniques. *Gastroenterology.* 1999;116(3):735-760.
6. Rao SS. Diagnosis and management of fecal incontinence. American College of Gastroenterology Practice Parameters Committee. *Am J Gastroenterol.* 2004;99(8):1585-1604.

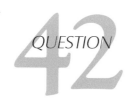

THE ADMITTING HOUSESTAFF CAN'T FIGURE OUT WHERE TO ADMIT PATIENTS WITH DIVERTICULITIS. WHAT CAN I TELL THEM ABOUT THIS CONDITION?

Inku Hwang, MD

Diverticulitis is the term used to describe inflammation/infection associated with diverticulosis. Diverticulosis, the presence of benign outpouchings of the gastrointestinal (most commonly colonic) lumen, is a common condition with a prevalence that increases with age, reaching approximately 65% by 85 years. Although most people with diverticulosis remain asymptomatic, complications such as diverticulitis or diverticular bleeding can occur in up to 25% of patients during their lifetime.[1,2]

Diverticulitis is thought to develop through the erosion or obstruction of a diverticular orifice by a fecolith or other stool debris, leading to bacterial proliferation, inflammation, and microperforation. This most commonly occurs in the left colon in Western countries and occurs in the right colon in only about 1.5% of cases, although this number is much higher in Asians.[3] Patients with diverticulitis usually present with left lower quadrant abdominal pain lasting for 24 hours or longer. Constipation, diarrhea, nausea, and vomiting can also occur, and dysuria, urinary urgency, and/or frequency is present in up to 15% of cases if the inflamed segment is near the urinary bladder or if there is a colovesicular fistula.[4,5] Up to 50% of patients with diverticulitis report a history of prior similar episodes. On physical exam, abdominal tenderness to palpation is often found, and in about 20% of cases, a tender mass may be felt.[1] If diverticulitis is complicated by gross peritoneal perforation and peritonitis, peritoneal signs should be seen, and amylase or lipase may be mildly elevated. Although fever with mild leukocytosis is common, in nearly 50% of cases, the white blood count can be normal.[6] Finally, although the diagnosis is often made by a thorough history and physical exam, an abdominal CT scan is helpful to confirm the diagnosis, determine the severity, and identify possible complications (Figure 42-1).

Figure 42-1. Abscess complicating diverticulitis is evident on this CT scan of the pelvis.

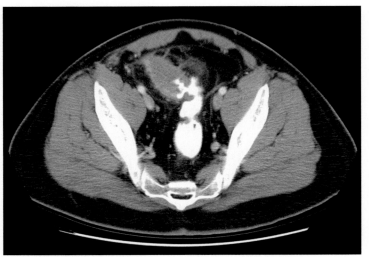

The first step for admitting housestaff is to determine whether the patient has complicated or uncomplicated diverticulitis. Those with complicated diverticulitis (ie, those with gross perforation with peritonitis, obstruction, abscess, or fistula formation) should be admitted for intravenous antibiotics and evaluation for surgical management. Those with uncomplicated diverticulitis may be managed as outpatients with oral antibiotics and close follow-up. Up to one-third of these patients may require subsequent surgical management. The issues to consider in determining whether the patient with uncomplicated diverticulitis can be managed as an outpatient include age, comorbidities, the ability to take oral medications, and the severity of presentation.[7] It is prudent to admit elderly patients for intravenous antibiotics who may not have adequate social support systems, who may have multiple comorbid conditions, and who may not be able to tolerate oral antibiotics.

It is important to realize that the probability of recurrent attacks increases with each episode of diverticulitis. Thus, a patient with 2 or more episodes of diverticulitis, especially if young and a good surgical candidate, should be considered for a partial colonic resection to prevent recurrences and subsequent complications. Also, it should be remembered that malignancy can mimic diverticulitis, and patients with an episode of diverticulitis who have not undergone colon cancer screening should be referred for colonoscopy after the antibiotic therapy has been completed and symptoms have resolved. Colonoscopy in the acute diverticulitis setting is not recommended as it associated with an increased risk of colonic perforation.

References

1. Parks TG. Natural history of diverticular disease of the colon. *Clin Gastroenterol.* 1975;4(1):53-69.
2. Painter NS, Burkitt DP. Diverticular disease of the colon, a 20th century problem. *Clin Gastroenterol.* 1975;4(1):3-21.
3. Fischer MG, Farkas AM. Diverticulitis of the cecum and ascending colon. *Dis Colon Rectum.* 1984;27(7):454-458.
4. Konvolinka CW. Acute diverticulitis under age forty. *Am J Surg.* 1994;167(6):562-565.

5. Ferzoco LB, Raptopoulos V, Silen W. Acute diverticulitis. *N Engl J Med.* 1998;338(21):1521-1526.

6. Ambrosetti P, Robert JH, Witzig JA, et al. Acute left colonic diverticulitis: a prospective analysis of 226 consecutive cases. *Surgery.* 1994;115(5):546-550.

7. Stollman NH, Raskin JB. Diagnosis and management of diverticular disease of the colon in adults. Ad Hoc Practice Parameters Committee of the American College of Gastroenterology. *Am J Gastroenterol.* 1999;94(11):3110-3121.

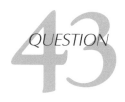

WHAT SHOULD BE MY RESPONSE TO PATIENTS WHO ASK ABOUT ANTIBIOTIC PROPHYLAXIS FOR THEIR COLONOSCOPIES? IF THEY ARE PERSISTENT, AND DO NOT HAVE AN INDICATION, IS IT OK TO ACQUIESCE?

Inku Hwang, MD

Gastrointestinal endoscopies are low-risk procedures for endocarditis or other infectious complications, and thus, for many of these procedures, including colonoscopies with and without biopsies, prophylactic antibiotics are generally not recommended. This is based on the low reported incidence of endocarditis and the lack of any clear benefit with prophylactic antibiotics. Adding to the arguments against antibiotic prophylaxis for colonoscopy are the facts that the bacteria that enter the blood during colonoscopy are not those typically associated with endocarditis, and the inappropriate use of antibiotics can cause resistant organisms and increase the risk of antibiotic-related complications.

Table 43-1 lists the guidelines for use of prophylactic antibiotics for endoscopy published by the American Society of Gastrointestinal Endoscopy (ASGE).[1]

In determining the need for prophylactic antibiotics, one must consider the patient's risk of infectious complications as well as the bacteremic potential of the endoscopic procedure being contemplated. Colonoscopies are considered low risk for bacteremia, and other than for a select group of high-risk patients undergoing high risk procedures (where antibiotics are considered optional), prophylactic antibiotics are not recommended with colonoscopy.

The American Heart Association (AHA) has published similar guidelines stratifying cardiac lesions with the risk of procedures.[2] Historically, the AHA guidelines have been

Table 43-1

Prophylaxis Recommendations for Patients Undergoing Endoscopic Procedures

Patient Condition	Procedure Contemplated	Antibiotic Prophylaxis
High Risk • Bile-duct obstruction in absence of cholangitis • Sterile pancreatic fluid collection • Cystic lesions along GI tract • All patients	• ERCP with anticipated incomplete drainage • ERCP or transmural drainage • EUS-FNA • Percutaneous endoscopic feeding tube placement; Cirrhosis with acute bleeding	Recommended
Insufficient Data • Solid lesion along the lower GI tract	• EUS-FNA	Prophylaxis optional
Low Risk • All cardiac conditions; synthetic vascular graft and other nonvalvular cardiovascular devices; prosthetic joints • Bile duct obstruction in the absence of cholangitis • Solid lesion along the lower GI tract	• Any endoscopic procedure • ERCP with complete drainage • EUS-FNA	Not indicated and/or not recommended

Cardiac prophylaxis regimens (oral 1 hr before, IM or IV 30 min before procedure)
Amoxicillin PO or Ampicillin IV: adult 2.0 g, child 50 mg/kg
Penicillin allergic: clindamycin (adult 600 mg, child 20 mg/kg), or cephalexin or cefadroxil (adults 2.0 g, child 50 mg/kg), or azithromycin, or clarithromycin (adult 500 mg, child 15 mg/kg), or cefazolin (adult 1.0 g, child 25 mg/kg IV or IM), or vancomycin (adult 1.0 g, child 10-20 mg/kg IV).

ERCP: endoscopic retrograde cholangiopancreatography; EUS-FNA: endoscopic ultrasound with fine needle aspiration; GI: gastrointestinal; IM: intramuscular; IV: intravenous

more stringent than those of the ASGE. In 2007, however, the AHA published new guidelines that represented a significant change from previous versions. For endoscopic practice, the AHA concluded that administration of prophylactic antibiotics solely to prevent IE is not recommended for patients who undergo gastrointestinal endoscopic procedures. Specifically, both the AHA and the ASGE state that prophylaxis against endocarditis is not recommended for colonoscopy or any other gastrointestinal endoscopy.[1,2] The recommendations for prophylaxis in Table 43-1 are geared toward preventing bacteremia and subsequent sepsis in patients with high-risk conditions that make them prone to disseminated infections.

So what do we tell the insistent patient who has been told to get antibiotics before any procedure? Perhaps the best course to take is to clarify the patient's cardiac condition, listen carefully to his or her concerns, and then educate him or her on why antibiotic prophylaxis is generally not used with colonoscopy. One must explain that endocarditis after colonoscopy is very rare and that the bacteria that generally cause endocarditis are not found in the colon. Also, the patient should be told that indiscriminate use of antibiotics can lead to resistance and complications, including *Clostridium difficile* colitis. Most patients respond well to this and will likely understand that the provider is doing his or her best for them.

References

1. Banerjee S, Shen B, Baron TH, et al. Antibiotic prophylaxis for GI endoscopy. *Gastrointest Endosc.* 2008;67(6):791-798.
2. Wilson W, Taubert KA, Gewitz M, et al. Prevention of infective endocarditis: guidelines from the American Heart Association: a guideline from the American Heart Association Rheumatic Fever, Endocarditis, and Kawasaki Disease Committee, Council on Cardiovascular Disease in the Young, and the Council on Clinical Cardiology, Council on Cardiovascular Surgery and Anesthesia, and the Quality of Care and Outcomes Research Interdisciplinary Working Group. *Circulation.* 2007;116(15):1736-1754.

THE DIABETES CLINIC WANTS A LECTURE ON THE EFFECTS OF DIABETES ON COLONIC MOTILITY. WHAT CAN I TELL THEM IN 5 MINUTES OR LESS?

Inku Hwang, MD

Diabetes is a systemic disorder, and its resultant neuropathy and vasculopathy can affect any organ in the body including those of the gastrointestinal tract. Although diabetic motility disorders of the upper gastrointestinal tract, such as diabetic gastroparesis, are well described, motility disorders affecting the colon, although common, are less well studied. Patients with diabetes and visceral neuropathy can have symptoms of constipation, diarrhea, fecal incontinence, and rarely steatorrhea due to several mechanisms.

Although the exact prevalence of constipation and diarrhea is difficult to determine, studies suggest that it is relatively common in diabetics. In one study, up to 29% of patients with at least 1 complication of diabetes also had constipation,[1] and diarrhea was found in 8% to 22% of diabetic patients.[2,3] Because most centers do not perform colonic motility studies (in contrast to the relatively accessible gastric emptying studies for gastroparesis), the exact mechanism of the colonic dysmotility seen with diabetes is unclear. It is likely that the visceral neuropathy from diabetes affects both the autonomic (vagus and sympathetic) and enteric nervous systems (submucosal and myenteric nerves), resulting in alteration of colonic and small bowel motility patterns. Dysregulation of the enteric nervous system resulting in abnormal transport of water and ions across the mucosa has also been implicated as a cause of the diarrhea seen in some diabetics.[4] Further complicating the picture, small bowel dysmotility may lead to bacterial overgrowth and subsequent bile salt deconjugation and steatorrhea. Finally, these patients are often on multiple medications, such as metformin, and they may be using artificial non-absorbed sweeteners, such as sorbitol, which can also result in diarrhea.[5,6]

Diabetic diarrhea is a unique entity typically found in patients with longstanding, advanced diabetes with other complications from chronic hyperglycemia. These patients classically present with intermittent bouts of watery diarrhea without pain or tenesmus, which may occur at night, and are intermixed with episodes of normal bowel habits. These episodes start and end suddenly, without any inciting etiologies or treatments. Up to 10% of diabetics also can be affected by incontinence due to decreased anorectal sensation, reduced resting sphincter pressures, and possibly altered compliance of the rectum.[7]

The general approach to diabetic patients with these symptoms involves adequate evaluation with a variety of laboratory and endoscopic tests designed to exclude other etiologies. The mainstay of therapy includes treatment of the underlying diabetes with tight glucose control, maintenance of normal electrolyte balance, correction of any nutritional deficiencies, and elimination of any medications that may cause or exacerbate the symptoms. Specific therapies include a trial of fiber to alter the consistency of stools, loperamide for diarrhea, and antibiotics if bacterial overgrowth is suspected. Also, for the patient with diabetic diarrhea, a trial of clonidine or octreotide may be beneficial.[4] Patients with fecal incontinence should undergo anorectal manometry to determine if biofeedback is an option (see Questions 13 and 41).

References

1. Bytzer P, Talley NJ, Hammer J, Young LJ, Jones MP, Horowitz M. GI symptoms in diabetes mellitus are associated with both poor glycemic control and diabetic complications. *Am J Gastroenterol.* 2002;97(3):604-611.
2. Dandona P, Fonseca V, Mier A, Beckett AG. Diarrhea and metformin in a diabetic clinic. *Diabetes Care.* 1983;6(5):472-474.
3. Feldman M, Schiller LR. Disorders of gastrointestinal motility associated with diabetes mellitus. *Ann Intern Med.* 1983;98(3):378-384.
4. Chang EB, Fedorak RN, Field M. Experimental diabetic diarrhea in rats. Intestinal mucosal denervation hypersensitivity and treatment with clonidine. *Gastroenterology.* 1986;91(3):564-569.
5. Bytzer P, Talley NJ, Jones MP, Horowitz M. Oral hypoglycaemic drugs and gastrointestinal symptoms in diabetes mellitus. *Aliment Pharmacol Ther.* 2001;15(1):137-142.
6. Badiga MS, Jain NK, Casanova C, Pitchumoni CS. Diarrhea in diabetics: the role of sorbitol. *J Am Coll Nutr.* 1990;9(6):578-582.
7. Wald A. Incontinence and anorectal dysfunction in patients with diabetes mellitus. *Eur J Gastroenterol Hepatol.* 1995;7(8):737-739.

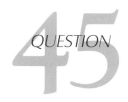

WHAT ARE THE ADVERSE EFFECTS OF NONSTEROIDAL ANTI-INFLAMMATORY DRUGS ON THE COLON AND HOW CAN THEY BE MITIGATED?

Scott L. Itzkowitz, DO, FACP

Nonsteroidal anti-inflammatory drugs (NSAIDs) are one of the most common classes of drugs taken by patients. Aside from the effects seen in the upper gastrointestinal tract (most notably the development of erosions or frank peptic ulcer disease), there are also several less well-known adverse effects in the colon. It could be argued that the increased use of enteric-coated or sustained-release preparations, in an attempt to decrease the gastroduodenal side effects of this class of medications, has shifted the potential for adverse events secondary to NSAIDs to the distal small intestine and colon. Although popular belief has been that NSAIDs cause negative effects due to localized mucosal injury (a fact supported by the occasional observation of NSAID capsules or tablets at the site of ulcers), a more likely mechanism is through the systemic inhibition of protective prostaglandins and COX-1. The inhibition of these protective factors leads to vasoconstriction and mucosal ischemia, which in turn promotes the release of proinflammatory cytokines and luminal factors, leading to subsequent mucosal damage manifested by mucosal inflammation and ulceration.[1]

The ileo-cecal region is the most common distal gastrointestinal site of potential NSAID-induced damage, and the NSAID effects observed in this region of the colon are similar to those in the upper gastrointestinal tract. Erosions, ulcers, and secondary complications of these mucosal lesions (perforation, strictures, formation of "diaphragms," obstruction) can be found in the region of the colon and have all been documented. NSAIDs have also been linked to the development of colitis with the disease ranging from limited disease in the rectum (proctitis) to pan-colitis. Symptoms most commonly encountered in patients with NSAID-induced colitis include diarrhea with or without hematochezia, which may mimic ulcerative colitis, which rapidly improves within days upon cessation of the offending NSAID. Histologic examination of the colon reveals a mild nonspecific colitis. Although the fenemates are the most notorious NSAID class associated with colitis, all NSAIDs have been implicated as etiologies of this complication. Initially, it was believed that because of the increase in production of prostaglandins, NSAIDs might actually have been beneficial in the treatment of ulcerative colitis. However, subsequent studies showed a detrimental effect from NSAIDs in patients with inflammatory bowel disease. It is now widely believed that NSAIDs may cause relapse of quiescent inflammatory bowel disease and should be avoided in these patients.[2] Additionally, it has been shown that NSAIDs may trigger or exacerbate microscopic colitis, particularly collagenous colitis.

There have been multiple reports of ulceration throughout the colon related to NSAID therapy. These ulcers can occur both with systemic therapy and locally from NSAIDs given rectally. Histologically, these ulcers are nonspecific and, therefore, may be hard to differentiate from idiopathic ulcers that are unrelated to NSAID therapy. NSAIDs are also thought to exacerbate lesions already present in the colon and, through their platelet inhibitory effects, may increase the risk of bleeding from diverticuli or arteriovenous malformations.

Although there is some evidence to suggest that the risk of developing serious lower gastrointestinal complications may be decreased with the utilization of selective COX-2 inhibitors, the major way of treating NSAID-induced complications is to discontinue therapy. Except for lesions involving chronic fibrotic strictures, the majority of complications (ulceration, colitis) improve promptly upon discontinuation of the NSAID. If symptoms do not resolve rapidly after stopping NSAID therapy, consider another etiology or the possibility of continued (perhaps inadvertent) NSAID usage.

References

1. Laine L, Connors LG, Reicin A, et al. Serious lower gastrointestinal clinical events with nonselective NSAID or coxib use. *Gastroenterology.* 2003;124:288-292.
2. Bjarnason I, Hayllar J, MacPherson A, Russell A. Side effects of non-steroidal anti-inflammatory drugs on the small and large intestine in humans. *Gastroenterology.* 1993;104(6):1832-1847.

WHEN DO I NEED TO REFER A PATIENT WITH DIVERTICULAR BLEEDING FOR A COLECTOMY AND WHAT TESTS SHOULD BE DONE BEFORE THIS HAPPENS?

Scott L. Itzkowitz, DO, FACP

Colonic diverticular bleeding is the most common cause of rapid hematochezia (maroon or bright red bleeding), accounting for approximately 42% of cases of massive gastrointestinal blood loss.[1] Although diverticulosis is very common, diverticular bleeding only occurs in about 15% patients with this condition. Approximately one-third of patients with diverticular bleeding will be classified as having massive bleeding.[2] Bleeding diverticuli are most often found in the right colon and rarely accompany diverticulitis, which is more common in the left colon. Approximately 50% of patients with diverticular bleeds have had a previous episode.

The pathophysiology of diverticular bleeding is directly linked to structural abnormalities and intracolonic pressures. Blood vessels that penetrate the area of colonic wall weakness that define diverticuli are thin walled. Repeated eversion of the diverticulum results in recurring injury that promotes further thinning of the vessel wall, leading to segmental weakness of the artery and eventual rupture into the lumen of the bowel.

The management of massive diverticular bleeding includes resuscitation and stabilization of the patient, localization and diagnosis of the bleeding site, and, if possible, endoscopic hemostasis. Early surgical consultation in patients with suspected diverticular bleeding is an important aspect of the care of these patients. Most diverticular bleeds are self-limited, but some patients will continue to exhibit lower gastrointestinal bleeding after resuscitation and colonic purging. The initial diagnostic procedure of choice is urgent colonoscopy, which should be performed within 6 to 12 hours of presentation.[3] If the culprit diverticulum is confidently identified at the time of colonoscopy through visualization of active bleeding (Figure 46-1), a nonbleeding visible vessel, or overlying

Figure 46-1. Actively bleeding colonic diverticulum prior to endoscopic therapy.

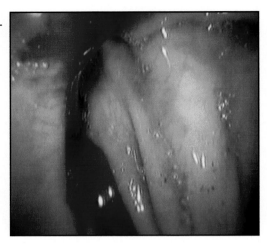

Figure 46-2. Bleeding diverticulum after endoscopic clipping.

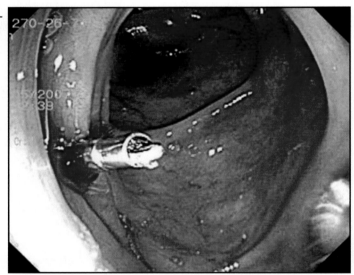

clot, endoscopic hemostasis can be performed by injecting 1:10,000 epinephrine in and around the vessel, applying bipolar coaptive coagulation to the incident vessel or both. Endoscopically deployed hemostatic clipping devices may also be used with success (Figure 46-2).

When a persistently bleeding lesion cannot be identified or controlled by endoscopic means, consideration should be given to performing angiography with or without prior nuclear imaging. Nuclear imaging utilizing either technetium 99 sulfur colloid or 99 m pertechnate can be used to identify active bleeding at a rate of at least 0.1 mL/min and is noninvasive. Nuclear imaging methods are limited, however, in that they are only able to localize bleeding to quadrants of the abdomen, and no therapeutic options exist with these techniques. Arteriography has high specificity for localization of incident lesions with bleeding rates greater than 0.5 mL/min and may be particularly useful when nuclear imaging is positive. Arteriography has the added benefit of allowing therapeutic intervention. Vasopressin infusion and embolization can be performed via this procedure, with successful cessation of bleeding in up to 91% of cases; however, as many as 50% will rebleed with cessation of vasopressin.[4] The potential complications of arteriography include arterial thrombosis with resultant intestinal infarction or renal failure. A relatively new technique, dynamic enhanced helical computed tomography, is less invasive than angiography but more accurate than nuclear imaging and has shown promise in initial studies for the diagnosis of sources of active lower gastrointestinal bleeding. These techniques also help to exclude bleeding sites in the proximal gastrointestinal tract.

Some patients will have massive diverticular bleeding that defies localization or endoscopic hemostasis, and surgical intervention is warranted in these instances. The majority of these cases occur in patients who have persistent hemodynamic instability in the face of aggressive resuscitation attempts. Exploratory laparotomy is considered the final diagnostic test, and a source is found in more than 75% of cases; these yields are increased further with intraoperative colonoscopy. If an incident lesion is localized, a segmental colectomy should be performed. For patients who continue to bleed without a documented site of bleeding, subtotal colectomy may be performed with low rates of rebleeding; however, the morbidity and mortality rates are significantly higher in these patients compared to those in which a source is identified.

References

1. Longstreth GF. Epidemiology and outcome of patients hospitalized with acute lower gastrointestinal hemorrhage. A population-based study. *Am J Gastroenterol.* 1997;92(3):419-424.
2. Imbembo AL, Bailey RW. Diverticular disease of the colon. In: Sabiston DC Jr, ed. *Textbook of Surgery.* 14th ed. Philadelphia, PA: Churchill Livingstone; 1992:910.
3. Jensen DM, Machicado GA, Jutabha R, Kovacs TO. Urgent colonoscopy for the diagnosis and treatment of severe diverticular hemorrhage. *N Engl J Med.* 2000;342(2):78-82.
4. Browder W, Cerise EJ, Litwin MS. Impact of emergency angiography in massive lower gastrointestinal bleeding. *Ann Surg.* 1986;204(5):530-536.

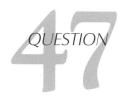
WHAT DO I TELL A PATIENT WHO I JUST DIAGNOSED WITH STAGE IIB COLON CANCER REGARDING TREATMENT AND PROGNOSIS?

Scott L. Itzkowitz, DO, FACP

Long-term treatment recommendations and prognosis of colon cancer are based on tumor stage at the time of initial diagnosis. Based on the TNM staging system, stage IIB cancer is any cancer considered T4 (tumor invades other organs or structures and/or perforates the visceral peritoneum) (Figure 47-1) without nodal or distant metastases (N0, M0). While initial clinical staging can be done through radiographic, endoscopic, and/or intraoperative means, pathologic staging serves as the basis for estimated survival rates. The current 5-year survival rate for stage IIB colon cancer is 72%.[1]

The only absolute means of cure for localized colon cancer is surgical resection. There are several goals at the time of surgery. The first is to thoroughly explore the abdomen to rule out extracolonic spread. Next, a complete resection of the involved bowel with the goal of achieving negative proximal, distal, and radial margins should be carried out. Adequate lymph node dissection is a crucial aspect of this procedure, and at least 12 lymph nodes should be harvested.[2] Restoration of the continuity of the bowel is always planned; however, the adequacy of the resection should never be sacrificed in attempts to prevent an ostomy. Cecal resections should include a segment of terminal ileum as well as its mesentery. Tumors in the ascending colon can be treated with a standard right hemicolectomy, while lesions at the hepatic flexure usually require an extended right hemicolectomy. Tumors in the mid-transverse colon require a resection from the hepatic flexure to the splenic flexure. Left colon cancers can either be resected with a left hemicolectomy or segmental colectomy as long as negative margins and adequate resection of draining lymphatics can be achieved. Although the majority of oncologic surgery for colon cancer is still done utilizing

Figure 47-1. Obstructing T4 cancer of the sigmoid colon.

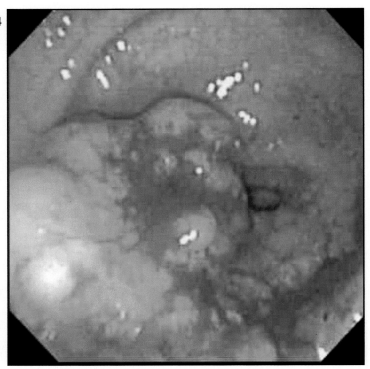

open surgery, laparoscopic colon resection (LCR) and hand-assisted LCR as curative surgery for colon cancer is evolving.

Although adjuvant chemotherapy for Stage III or greater colon cancer utilizing 5-FU/leucovorin regimens is considered standard, data do not currently support its use in most cases of Stage II disease. The American Society of Clinical Oncology guidelines currently only recommend chemotherapy for patients with Stage II colon cancer if the lymph node resection was inadequate, if the lesion is T4, if there is evidence of perforation, or if the histology shows the lesion to be poorly differentiated, although there is a paucity of clinical trial data to support these recommendations.

References

1. O'Connell JB, Maggard MA, Ko CY. Colon cancer survival rates with the new American Joint Committee on Cancer sixth edition staging. *J Natl Cancer Inst.* 2004;96(19):1420-1425.
2. Baxter NN, Virnig DJ, Rothenberger DA, Morris AM, Jessurun J, Virnig BA. Lymph node evaluation in colorectal cancer patients: a population-based study. *J Natl Cancer Inst.* 2005;97(3):219-225.

THE WARD TEAM HAS A PATIENT WITH A DISTENDED ABDOMEN AND INCREASING GAS-FILLED LOOPS OF BOWEL ON X-RAY. HOW CAN I HELP THEM RECOGNIZE AND TREAT COLONIC PSEUDO-OBSTRUCTION (OGILVIE'S SYNDROME)?

Scott L. Itzkowitz, DO, FACP

Acute colonic pseudo-obstruction (Ogilvie's syndrome) is characterized by dilation of the right colon and cecum not caused by a luminal obstructive lesion. Although Ogilvie's syndrome was classically described as being related to an underlying retroperitoneal malignancy, today the term is used to describe acute pseudo-obstruction related to any cause. The 3 most common etiologies include trauma, infection, and cardiovascular disease, but patients with systemic illnesses can also develop Ogilvie's.[1] The actual mechanism of the disorder is unknown, but it is believed that some abnormality affecting the autonomic nervous system might be involved. It is more common in men, particularly in patients who are older than 60 years.

Clinically, patients present with significant abdominal distention, which may be associated with nausea, vomiting, abdominal pain, constipation, and occasionally diarrhea. There are no specific physical or laboratory findings. On physical examination, bowel sounds are present, and abdominal tympany can be elicited in most patients. Peritoneal signs are usually absent, but if they are present, such findings suggest impending perforation. Clinicians should exclude electrolyte abnormalities, such as hypokalemia, hypocalcemia, or hypomagnesemia. Leukocytosis should not be seen with uncomplicated acute pseudo-obstruction. Radiologic studies such as plain or upright abdominal radiographs

Figure 48-1. Colonic pseudo-obstruction.

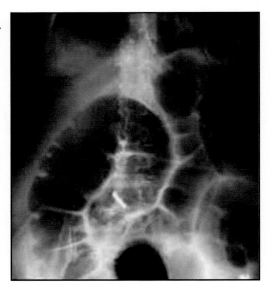

will reveal a significantly dilated colon, usually from the cecum to the splenic flexure, but occasionally all the way to the rectum, with normal haustral markings (Figure 48-1). The diagnosis of Ogilvie's syndrome should be entertained only after toxic megacolon or mechanical obstruction is ruled out. If patients appear systemically ill with fever, tachycardia, or significant abdominal tenderness, one should consider the possibility of toxic megacolon. If there is any suspicion of mechanical obstruction, a water-soluble contrast enema of the rectum and distal colon should be performed. Besides the diagnostic yield, this maneuver has the added benefit of stimulating colonic motility and may potentially improve symptoms in acute pseudo-obstruction.

Treatment recommendations are based mainly on anecdotal experience and retrospective reviews because there are few controlled therapeutic trials of Ogilvie's syndrome. Initial treatment should be based on the remediation of potential secondary causes of colonic atony, such as narcotic medications. Any underlying electrolyte abnormalities should be corrected, and attempts at mobilization of bed-bound patients should be undertaken. In patients who are symptomatic without significant colonic dilation (usually defined as a cecal diameter of >12 cm), consideration should also be given to alternating body position, nasogastric tube decompression, and/or placement of a rectal tube (with or without serial tap water enemas). These conservative measures should be used for 24 to 48 hours while obtaining serial abdominal x-rays and routine labs every 12 to 24 hours.

If patients develop increasing abdominal pain or peritoneal signs, or if abdominal cecal diameter exceeds 12 cm, advanced treatment should ensue. Neostigmine 2.0 mg IV, up to 2 doses, has shown a marked durable response, which usually occurs in minutes in controlled trials. Neostigmine should be given in a monitored environment with atropine at the bedside due to the potential for this agent to incite clinically significant bradycardia. In patients who are not judged to be neostigmine candidates or those who fail this therapy, unprepped colonoscopic decompression with or without the placement of a decompression tube should be performed. For patients who ultimately fail medical or endoscopic therapy, surgical management with cecostomy or colectomy may be considered. Percutaneous cecostomy may also be an option for recalcitrant patients with acute colonic pseudo-obstruction.[2,3]

References

1. Vanek VW, Al-Salti M. Acute pseudo-obstruction of the colon (Ogilvie's syndrome). An analysis of 400 cases. *Dis Colon Rectum.* 1986;29(3):203-210.
2. Eisen GM, Baron TH, Dominitz JA, et al. Acute colonic pseudo-obstruction. *Gastrointest Endosc.* 2002;56(6): 789-792.
3. McConnell EJ, Pemberton JH. *Sleisenger and Fordtran's Gastrointestinal and Liver Disease.* 7th ed. Philadelphia, PA: Saunders; 2002:2137-2138.

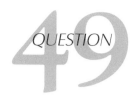

WHAT ARE THE VARIOUS MANIFESTATIONS OF E. COLI INFECTION OF THE COLON AND HOW SHOULD IT BE TREATED?

Scott L. Itzkowitz, DO, FACP

Escherichia coli (E. coli) is a common commensal organism of the gastrointestinal tract. However, when specific additional genes are acquired by these bacteria, they may become pathogenic, and *E. coli* represents one of the most common bacterial causes of diarrheal illness in humans. There are 5 specific forms of *E. coli* that are clinically relevant: enterotoxigenic *E. coli* (ETEC), enteropathogenic *E. coli* (EPEC), enterohemorrhagic *E. coli* (EHEC), enteroinvasive *E. coli* (EIEC), and enteroaggregative *E. coli* (EAEC). The pathogenic *E. coli* cannot be distinguished from nonpathogenic strains by culture or routine biochemical testing, and additional testing must be performed. Currently, EHEC O157 is the only pathogenic strain readily identified in the clinical laboratory; further testing is currently only performed in research laboratories.[1,2]

ETEC has emerged as a significant pathogen in the United States and elsewhere. It is a fastidious organism and is commonly found in food and water supplies, particularly in developing nations. It is one of the most common bacterial causes of diarrheal illness in children younger than 2 years of age and is the most frequent cause of "traveler's diarrhea." After exposure, the patient usually experiences watery diarrhea, which may be very similar to cholera with some nausea. Vomiting is uncommon. Usually the illness lasts less than 24 hours, but can persist for up to 4 or 5 days. Currently, the diagnosis is only performed in research laboratories. Treatment consists primarily of oral rehydration. In most cases, the disease is self-limited, and antimicrobial therapy is usually not necessary. If treatment is necessary, consideration may be given for ciprofloxacin or a nonabsorbed gut-specific antibiotic, such as rifaximin.

EPEC primarily causes diarrhea in children, particularly neonates, and is an uncommon cause of clinical symptoms in adults. The diarrheal illness induced by EPEC can be extremely severe with vomiting and associated dehydration and malnutrition. Current means of diagnosis requires a deoxyribonucleic acid probe or polymerase chain reaction of the EPEC adherence factor and is performed only in research laboratories. Therapy consists of supportive care with rehydration.

As its name would imply, EHEC has been associated with outbreaks of bloody diarrhea. The production of one or more pathogenic Shiga toxins (of which O157:H7 is the most prevalent) by EHEC differentiates this organism from other *E. coli* species and is associated with an increased incidence of serious complications. Although infected beef is the most likely vector, ingestion of contaminated milk, drinking water, fruits, and vegetables has been isolated as a source of epidemics with EHEC. Once exposed, the incubation period is between 3 and 4 days. In addition to causing colitis, EHEC is also associated with hemolytic-uremic syndrome (HUS), primarily in children under age 10 and the elderly. HUS is characterized by the triad of acute renal failure, microangiopathic hemolytic anemia, and thrombocytopenia. EHEC should be considered in any patient who presents with bloody diarrhea, particularly in the setting of prominent abdominal pain without fever.[3] Diagnosis is made by stool culture with specific testing for O157:H7 on sorbitol-MacConkey agar. Sorbitol negative colonies that are confirmed as *E. coli* are subsequently tested to see if they react with antiserum to O157 antigen. The only treatment of EHEC is supportive care with monitoring for the complications of HUS. Antibiotic therapy is not recommended due to the risk of increased production or release of toxin. In patients with HUS, consideration may be given for other therapies including plasma exchange, plasma infusion, or intravenous immunoglobulin, although these are of uncertain benefit.

EIEC causes a diarrhea that is very similar to shigellosis—watery and often associated with fever and abdominal cramping. The diarrhea associated with EIEC may occasionally be bloody. With an incubation period of less than 24 hours, EIEC contains adherence factors that allow it to invade enterocytes where it can multiply and move to adjacent intestinal cells. A definitive diagnosis can be made by stool culture with DNA probe searching for EIEC. Treatment is usually supportive with the goal of rehydration. In advanced cases, antimicrobial therapy with trimethoprim-sulfamethoxazole may be utilized.

EAEC causes persistent watery diarrhea usually in children, primarily in developing countries, though outbreaks have been reported in Europe and cases have been reported in HIV-infected adults. The complete pathogenesis of EAEC is not completely understood. Diagnosis is made by identification of a tissue adherence factor and is only performed in research laboratories. Successful treatment and eradication can be achieved via treatment with ciprofloxacin.

References

1. Nataro JP, Kaper JB. Diarrheagenic Escherichia coli. *Clin Microbiol Rev.* 1998;11(1):142-201.
2. March SB, Ratnam S. Sorbitol-MacConkey medium for detection of Escherichia coli O157:H7 associated with hemorrhagic colitis. *J Clin Microbiol.* 1986;23(5):869-872.
3. Boyce TG, Swerdlow DL, Griffin PM. Escherichia coli O157:H7 and the hemolytic-uremic syndrome. *N Engl J Med.* 1995;333(6):364-368.

INDEX

abdominal distention, in Ogilvie's syndrome, 177–179
acetylcholine, in colonic motility, 71–73
acid steatocrit, 99
adenocarcinoma
    rectal, 141–142
    recurrent, 38
adenoma
    serrated
        endoscopic appearance and histology of, 42
        features of, 39
        follow-up for, 40–43
        malignant potential of, 40–41
        neoplastic progression of, 42
        types of, 39–40
    serrated sessile, 39–40, 43
        management of, 41–42
        potential neoplastic progression of, 45–46
    tubular, surveillance after removal of, 23–25
adenoma-carcinoma sequence, 40–41
African American men, screening colonoscopy in, 3–4
AIDS, colonic infections associated with, 83–84
allopurinol, 134
aloe laxative, 51
alosetron
    contraindications to, 102
    for irritable bowel syndrome with diarrhea (IBS-D), 101–103
American Cancer Society Colorectal Cancer Advisory Committee guidelines, 35
American Heart Association, endoscopy cardiac risk guidelines of, 163–165
5-aminosalicylates
    for collagenous colitis, 109
    for pouchitis, 134
amoxicillin/clavulanate, 134
anal canal, 129
    pressures on in hemorrhoids, 129–130
anal fissures
    causes and characteristics of, 119
    incidence and prevalence of, 119
    management and treatment of, 119–121
    in pruritus ani, 125

in solitary rectal ulcer syndrome, 144
anal infections, in solitary rectal ulcer syndrome, 144
anal skin tags, 120
    in pruritus ani, 125
anal sphincters
    control of, 71–72
    division of, 120–121
    in fecal continence, 155
    high amplitude propagated contractions (HAPC), 72
    low amplitude propagated contractions (LAPC), 71–72
    spasms of, 119
angiography, for diverticular bleeding, 172–173
anorectal trauma, 143–144
anoscopy, 130
anthraquinone laxatives
    in colorectal cancer risk, 58
    in melanosis coli, 51–53
    neuropathic changes from, 77
antibiotics
    for bacterial overgrowth with diabetes, 168
    for *Clostridium difficile* in IBD flare, 95–97
    for collagenous colitis, 109
    for Escherichia coli infections, 182
    for irritable bowel syndrome, 91–93
    for pouchitis, 134
    prophylactic during colonoscopies, 163–165
antidiarrheals, 109
antihistamines, for pruritus ani, 125
antisecretory agents, 109
antispasmodics, for proctalgia fugax, 128
APC mutations, 46
argon plasma coagulation, 139
arteriography, for diverticular bleeding, 172–173
5-ASAs, for chemoprevention of colon cancer, 31
aspirin, prophylactic for colorectal cancer, 11–13
azathioprine, 110

backwash ileitis, 31
bacterial overgrowth
    with diabetes, 168
    in irritable bowel syndrome, 91–93